How to Communicate Effectively

in Health and Social Care

A practical guide
for the caring professions

Moi Ali

Pavilion

How to Communicate Effectively in Health and Social Care

A practical guide for the caring professions

© Moi Ali 2017

The author has asserted their right in accordance with the Copyright, Designs and Patents Act (1988) to be identified as the author of this work.

Published by:
Pavilion Publishing and Media Ltd
Rayford House
School Road
Hove
East Sussex
BN3 5HX
Tel: 01273 434 943
Fax: 01273 227 308
Email: info@pavpub.com

Published 2017

A catalogue record for this book is available from the British Library.

ISBN: 978-1-911028-37-6
EPDF: 978-1-910366-18-9

Pavilion is the leading training and development provider and publisher in the health, social care and allied fields, providing a range of innovative training solutions underpinned by sound research and professional values. We aim to put our customers first, through excellent customer service and value.

Author: Moi Ali
Production editor: Ruth Chalmers, Pavilion Publishing and Media Ltd
Cover design: Phil Morash, Pavilion Publishing and Media Ltd
Page layout and typesetting: Phil Morash, Pavilion Publishing and Media Ltd
Printing: CPI Anthony Rowe Ltd

Contents

About the author

Moi Ali is a communications consultant with over three decades' experience. During that time, she has acted as communications advisor to a number of NHS hospitals and healthcare clinics, to two children's hospices, a voluntary-sector hospital, the Royal College of Nursing in Scotland, and to healthcare charities. She is also founder of healthcare pressure group Good Practice, which campaigned to make family doctors more accountable.

Moi is a former vice president of the Nursing and Midwifery Council, the world's largest healthcare regulator. She served on the board of a large health authority, and is the former chair of a healthcare charity/social enterprise. Currently she is a member of the Board of the Scottish Ambulance Service, where she chairs the clinical governance committee. She also sits on the Board of the Professional Standards Authority for Health and Social Care.

She is a professional writer, specialising in communications – and she runs tailor-made communications programmes for organisations. She has written best-selling books for publishers such as Dorling Kindersley, Kogan Page and Heinemann, and has been published in *Health Service Journal* and *Quality in Primary Care*.

A week-long stay in hospital convinced Moi of the need for this book. She witnessed poor practitioner communication leading to misunderstanding, heightened anxiety for patients, and general unhappiness on the wards. Much of the communication was unintentional, yet there were occasions when it had a damaging effect. She realised that small, simple but important changes in the communications approach and behaviour by healthcare professionals could potentially lead to a greatly enhanced patient experience and clinical outcome, and to happier, more confident staff.

Acknowledgements

I am grateful to Dr Francis Tierney, Dr Paul Wilson OBE and David Hume for their comments on my manuscript. Thanks also to the excellent Health Management Library in Edinburgh for their assistance with a literature search and the supply of research papers and journals.

Foreword

Professor JG Cowpe, Emeritus Professor at Cardiff University, Consultant Oral Surgeon

Communication provides the cornerstone for healthcare provision by building a trusting relationship between healthcare staff and their patients. It contributes to patients feeling a sense of shared ownership of their own health and well-being. This is something which healthcare staff and patients should strive to achieve on a daily basis.

This user-friendly handbook provides useful guidance to all those who work in healthcare, whether clinicians or support staff, at any level of experience and expertise. As well as helping clinicians to add value to patient care through effective communication, this book is also a useful resource in undergraduate and postgraduate education and training. Lifelong learning, achieved through continuing personal and professional development (CPPD), is crucial to all those involved in healthcare provision. Building on the art of communication skills, as part of CPPD, contributes to a seamless transition throughout one's career. This handbook is also of practical value to healthcare colleagues working across the EU and beyond, taking into account the variances in service configuration and national standards across different countries. Communication between peers, allied professionals, patients and their families (and carers) contributes to the successful recovery of a patient through shared ownership of their health.

Interprofessional training, education and health service delivery is paramount. The patient voice and patient involvement in their own care is high on the agenda. Moi Ali's book supports these initiatives.

This book provides a variety of excellent guidance through theory, evidence-base, references and footnotes. The boxes, which feature throughout the handbook – including true stories, bullet-pointed checklists and reflections, along with the diagrams/figures – provide a valuable and easy-to-use toolkit to support effective communication.

Having worked in dental clinical academia and provided oral healthcare services over many years, I would recommend this very useful handbook to dental clinicians, dentists and dental care professionals, and to their support staff – and to anyone working in other branches of healthcare and social care. I would also highly recommend it for use across the breadth of undergraduate and postgraduate education and training.

To Eileen Ali, my mother,
who died while I was writing this book.

Is this book for you?

This practical, readable and accessible handbook is for anyone working in health and social care – from students undergoing professional education or on practice placements to recently qualified doctors, nurses, midwives and paramedics. Senior members of healthcare teams whose formal training may not have covered communications will find it helpful, as will many other staff, including non-regulated health and social care workers such as healthcare assistants, who have received limited formal training in communications.

The book will also be of value to non-clinical front-line staff who have contact with patients[1] and their families, whether in hospitals and clinics, doctors' and dentists' surgeries, pharmacies, residential care homes and day centres, and other community healthcare and social care settings.

Even those with no face-to-face patient contact at all, such as administrative staff who write to patients, deal with telephone enquiries or handle complaints, will gain much from the advice in this book on effective communication.

Overseas practitioners coming to work in the UK will also find this to be a practical resource, using it to improve their communication skills and understand the different cultural and communications expectations here in the UK. (Unlike a number of communications titles, this one is based largely upon British research findings.)

It also has value for readers looking for a post-qualification continuing professional development (CPD) communications refresher. The General Medical Council (GMC) publication *The State of Medical Education and Practice in the UK*[2] states that 'never before have good communication skills been so vital', and they go on to show how lack of effective communication with patients, and poor or non-existent sharing of information with colleagues, has led to a significant number of formal complaints about doctors. The GMC frequently lists communication as one of its top three concerns in the area of fitness to practise. Recurring issues include failure to meet communication needs, to provide appropriate information to patients and to listen; failure to provide or share

---

1   Throughout this book, the term 'patient' is used as a short-hand for the wide range of therapeutic relationships practitioners have with those using their professional services – who may be known as service users, clients, patients, or by some other term.

2   General Medical Council, (2011) *The State of Medical Education and Practice in the UK*. Available at: http://www.gmc-uk.org/State_of_medicine_Final_web.pdf_44213427.pdf (accessed February 2017).

information; and poor communication with young people. A third of complaints about GPs in 2013 concerned communication failure. The number of fitness-to-practise enquiries to the GMC increased from 5,168 in 2007 to 10,347 in 2012. Research by Plymouth University Medical School into these complaints in 2014[3] concluded: '[A]n increasing proportion of complaints are focused on issues involving communication.' The GMC's findings serve to remind us that across healthcare and social care, qualified practitioners still need to pay attention to communication throughout their careers.

There are books aimed at particular healthcare professional groups, most of them specific to a single profession, such as nurses or doctors. This book crosses the various professional boundaries in healthcare, providing communications advice that applies to the whole multidisciplinary team. Some publications are overly theoretical and written in a 'heavy' academic style that can be difficult to dip into. Although drawing on communications theory, this book is a practical, plain English, readable guide. It uses real-life examples, as well as opportunities for personal reflection, to encourage you to focus on and to improve your own communication skills. There are checklists, bullet-pointed dos and don'ts, and other devices to make this an accessible and useable handbook rather than a weighty academic tome.

Health authorities, NHS trusts and health boards are increasingly paying attention to the need to improve the patient experience and are seeing patient satisfaction as a good measure of overall performance. Where communication between patients and clinicians has been good, and where communication between clinicians is effective, the patient experience is significantly improved. Good communication is also key to building a positive and therapeutic relationship with patients. Clinical effectiveness is improved when there is confidence by patients in those who are providing care for them. Without effective communication, that relationship cannot be therapeutic. This book links effective communication with patient experience and therapeutic outcomes.

So is this book for you? It will make valuable reading for anyone wanting to improve their communication skills, whether dealing with customers over the counter in a high-street pharmacy, working in a busy NHS ward, private care home, voluntary-sector day centre or GP practice; ferrying patients to hospital in an ambulance; seeing service users one-to-one; or visiting clients in their homes. If you work in health or social care, at whatever level, the answer is yes – this book is for you!

---

3   Archer J, Regan de Bere S, Bryce M, Nunn S, Lynne N, Coombes L & Roberts M (2014) *Understanding the Rise in Fitness to Practise Complaints from Members of the Public*. Camera with Plymouth University.

Introduction

There was once a time when having adequate technical skills and competencies, and the appropriate clinical management plan, was sufficient to be considered an effective member of the healthcare team. A decent understanding of anatomy, disease and conditions was enough to make the grade. So-called 'bedside manner' was an optional extra that was often in short supply. However, as early as the 1960s the role of good communication in healthcare was recognised, and since the 1980s there has been a growing acceptance that effective communication is an essential skill for healthcare practitioners. A substantial body of research, some of which you can read about in subsequent chapters, has demonstrated how good communication can help produce positive patient outcomes. 'Good communication is critical to good healthcare,' says a 2016 publication by cancer charity Marie Curie.[4]

Today, effective communication is regarded as an essential skill for any healthcare or social care professional. For many years it has been a mandatory competency for those training as regulated healthcare professionals in the UK. The various healthcare professional codes of practice all demand good communication as a basic requirement.

Yet despite more than three decades' mainstream acceptance of the positive impact of good communication, and widespread understanding of the consequences of poor communication, first-class communication is not always evident on hospital wards, in doctors and dentists surgeries, in ambulances and at clinics. The Marie Curie paper cited above says that, even in 2016, 'inadequacies in communication are still damaging medical care and wasting much-needed NHS resources … [This paper] argues that we already have many of the tools we need to make inroads into the problem. And to do so without adding to NHS costs. What we have lacked is the will to stay the course in driving through the cultural change'.

Much lip-service has been paid to effective communication, but we cannot assume that every 21st century healthcare professional can or will, on every occasion, confidently employ a range of communications techniques to put patients[5]

---

4   McDonald A (2016) *A Long and Winding Road: Improving communication with patients in the NHS*. Available at: https://www.mariecurie.org.uk/globalassets/media/documents/policy/campaigns/the-long-and-winding-road.pdf (accessed February 2017).

5   The terms 'patient', 'client' and 'service user' are used interchangeably, although I recognise that many health and social care professionals will have only patients, or only service users. Please substitute my term for whatever expression is used in your own professional arena.

at ease to build rapport; to educate and inform clients; and to assist them in reaching shared decisions – all in turn boosting the likelihood of a positive patient experience. If that were so, grumbles about poor communication would not regularly feature in the top three causes of complaint about the NHS.

It has been found that even where the clinical care provided has been first class, poor communication can undermine what could have been a positive experience, leading to complaints and even legal action. An American report[6] found that '[e]ven surgeons with exemplary technical skills are vulnerable to allegations of malpractice if they mismanage the communication of critical information'. It continues:

> 'Analysis of more than 7,500 surgery-related malpractice cases finds that 26 percent involved significant communication errors. In more than half of these cases, the surgical technique was not questioned, but the patient's care was impacted by miscommunication within the surgical team – or more commonly, by inadequate communication with the patient.'

The late Kate Granger, a doctor with terminal cancer, and founder of the #hellomynameis campaign, wrote on the www.hellomynameis.org.uk website: 'I made the stark observation that many staff looking after me did not introduce themselves before delivering my care. It felt incredibly wrong that such a basic step in communication was missing'. It is indeed shocking that something as simple as an introduction should be overlooked, but it serves to underline how even the most common and basic communication ritual – saying hello – is not always observed by busy healthcare staff. The ability to communicate well should not be regarded as an innate skill that we all possess, as evidenced by Dr Granger's somewhat wanting experience. Establishing a relationship from the outset, starting with a friendly greeting, can set the tone and make future communication easier – or if this doesn't happen, make it harder. We all know that, yet somehow it doesn't always happen.

From an early age most of us learn to speak, to listen, to convey our feelings verbally and non-verbally, to read and to write. Communication is automatic, barely requiring any thought. We see someone we know and we speak to them almost as an automatic response, in a natural and usually fluent fashion. But does that mean we're good communicators? Good communication may come naturally to some, but the rest have to learn. Let this book be your guide.

---

6   CRICO Strategies (2015) *Malpractice Risks in Communication Failures 2015 Annual Benchmarking Report*. Available at: https://www.rmf.harvard.edu/Malpractice-Data/Annual-Benchmark-Reports/1-Request-CBS-Report-PDFs (accessed February 2017). (CRICO is a division of The Risk Management Foundation of the Harvard Medical Institutions, Incorporated.)

Read about the practical application of evidence-based techniques that will lead to real improvements in the way that you communicate with service users and colleagues. The guidance offered has a sound theoretical basis, but this is not an academic study of the theory of communication. References and notes have been kept to a minimum. Instead, true stories bring the subject to life. Arguably the stories are mere anecdotes, but they do reflect the reality of typical patient experiences. (The boxes labelled 'True Story' are real-life examples, albeit with details changed where necessary to protect anonymity. 'Typical Example' boxes are not based on specific cases, but are representative of the experiences of patients in health and social care settings.) Bullet-pointed checklists will assist you in implementing improvements in the way that you tackle communication. Throughout the book there is ample opportunity to reflect on your own practice. I hope that it will inspire you to think about how you communicate and to strive to be a better communicator.

Chapter 1: Communication and why effective communication is important

This introductory chapter provides an overview of the subject, explains what is meant by effective communication, and highlights the benefits it brings. It also explores the effects of poor communication. The chapter ends with a questionnaire designed to help you identify and reflect upon your own communication style, your strengths and your weaknesses.

One of the things that makes human beings different from other mammals is our ability to employ profoundly sophisticated ways of communicating and interacting with each other: we use language, for example. To be more precise, humans communicate in around 6,900[7] languages, depending on whether you count extinct ones and how you classify certain dialects. Professor David Crystal, Honorary Professor of Linguistics at the University of Wales in Bangor, says that his latest estimate, allowing for the fact that endangered languages are dying at the rate of about one every fortnight, is around 6,000 – not including braille, the various sign languages such as British Sign Language for people with hearing impairment, or the many computer programming languages that exist. Whichever figure you choose, it's a kaleidoscopic array, and when mixed with the bewildering diversity of cultures, and non-verbal expression, the clear transmission of information, emotion and care between people can become a complex process.

---

7   Crystal D (2010) *The Cambridge Encyclopaedia of Language* (3rd edition). Cambridge: Cambridge University Press.

So, having the ability to speak doesn't automatically make humans good communicators. The speaking part of effective communication is but one component. But let's start at the beginning, with a definition. 'Information is the currency of safe care, and communication is the vehicle by which that currency moves,' stated one report[8] on healthcare communication. It's a neat description, but as for a definition, communication is the imparting or exchange of information, thoughts or ideas using speech, writing, or some other medium such as signals or behaviour. At its most simple level, the communications process can be seen in the flowchart in Figure 1.1, which shows what happens in effective communication. A message is transmitted and received as intended.

Figure 1.1: Effective communication

> **Intended message:** an idea or information in your head that you want to share

> **Transmitted message:** your idea translated into spoken or written words

> **Received message:** the idea/information as heard/read by the recipient coincides with what you intended to communicate

The flowchart makes communication look easy, but we know from experience that it's more complicated than that. People are not merely radio transmitters, broadcasting audible messages in one direction. Nor are we like televisions, transmitting audio-visual messages in one direction (although we do convey visual messages when we speak). We are more like telephones, both transmitting and receiving – or perhaps the Skype analogy is better, where there is a visual communication element too. There is a speaker (transmitter) and a listener (receiver). In spoken communication, the speaker will by turn become the listener and vice versa. The recipient in the flowchart above will respond to the communication they have received, thus beginning the process all over again in the other direction. The telephone analogy does not end there. Like a phone, humans have an earpiece as well as a mouthpiece, because listening is a vital component of effective communication. (Read more about effective listening skills in Chapter 4.)

Unlike the simplistic flow chart above, real-life communication is less linear and more dynamic and complex, with multiple opportunities for things to go awry –

---

8   CRICO Strategies (2015) *Malpractice Risks in Communication Failures 2015 Annual Benchmarking Report*. Available at: https://www.rmf.harvard.edu/Malpractice-Data/Annual-Benchmark-Reports/1-Request-CBS-Report-PDFs (accessed February 2017).

especially in a healthcare setting. Figure 1.2 illustrates just a few of the hazards waiting to trip up practitioners as we try to communicate with others. Chapters 2 and 3 go into more detail about these and the many other factors that can interfere with the successful delivery of our messages.

Figure 1.2: Communication hazards

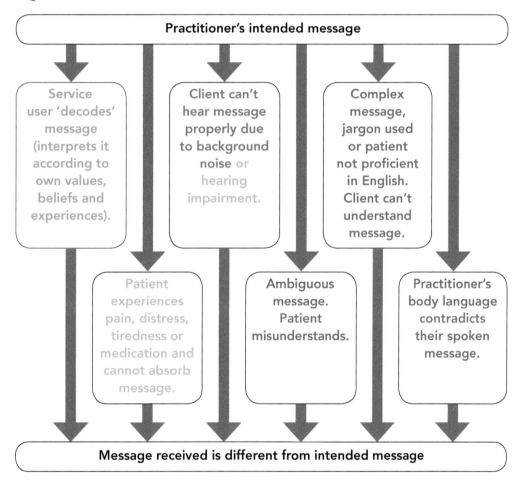

Key

- **Patient 'belief' factors:** A patient's previous experiences or their attitudes cause them to reframe your message to fit their specific beliefs.
- **Patient condition factors:** Your message is not absorbed due to the patient's condition (such as shock, medication, or dementia).
- **Environmental factors:** External factors such as noise interfere with the patient's ability to receive your message.
- **Practitioner factors:** You have not phrased your message in a way that can be understood by the patient, or your body language leads the patient to receive an unintended message from you.

Sometimes when communication goes wrong, the 'failure' lies with the practitioner – for example, when their message is over-complex or ambiguous and cannot be understood. However, this is not about apportioning blame; rather it is about learning from mistakes and improving practice. Even in situations where it is not the practitioner's 'fault', there may be things they could have done to improve the chances that their message would be received as intended – such as making environmental changes (reducing the volume on the TV in the nursing home) – or recognising the patient's condition and delaying communication until medication had worn off, or changing the style of communication to make it suitable for someone with a learning disability.

Not everything is within the control of the healthcare practitioner, though. Patients sometimes undertake biased or selective processing: to put it plainly, they hear what they want to hear. (That is something that humans in general can be prone to.) If the practitioner's message ('Substantially cut down on sweets and stop eating them altogether between meals to avoid further dental cavities') is one that the patient does not want to receive, they may subconsciously reframe it or over-simplify it ('If I eat sweets at meal times, I won't need fillings').

When your message fails to land as planned, understanding where it went wrong and why can help you to rephrase it so that it is understood. In the above example, there may be value in asking the patient to 'teach back' – a technique in which the healthcare practitioner checks they have been understood by asking the patient to summarise in their own words what has been said. 'When doing this, doctors should emphasise that what they are checking is their own ability to communicate, not the patient's ability to understand,' advises the Royal College of General Practitioners.[9] This technique also serves to improve patient recall, so they are more likely to remember what they have been told in a consultation.

Example 1.1 below shows a typical way that a message can go awry. Example 1.2 illustrates how a simple change to the message can avert the problem.

Example1.1

Intended message: The doctor would like to see you to discuss your test results.

Received message: Doctors only ask to see you to discuss results if it's serious, so I must be seriously ill. The doctor wants to see me face-to-face to break the bad news.

---

9   Royal College of General Practitioners (2014) *Health Literacy: Report from an RCGP-led health literacy workshop*. Available at: http://www.rcgp.org.uk/clinical-and-research/clinical-resources/health-literacy-report.aspx (accessed February 2017).

This straightforward factual request to see a patient has caused the patient needless fear and alarm. Anticipate how your message may be received, and amend it so as to avert potential misunderstanding. Put yourself in the patient's shoes and try to imagine how you – or someone close to you, such as your mother or grandfather – might react to your message. The interaction below shows how to do this.

Example 1.2

Intended message: The doctor would like to see you to discuss your test results.

Anticipated patient reaction: S/he may be worried about the results and fear the worst if asked to come to the surgery/clinic.

Rephrased message: The doctor would like to see you to discuss your test results, but it's normal practice to be asked to come into the surgery for this and there's nothing to worry about.

It really can be as simple as that. A reassuring few words and explanation can sometimes avert the kind of worry that could have harmful effects on a patient's well-being.

Why practitioners communicate

There are many reasons why practitioners and other healthcare staff need to communicate at work. They include:

- To *impart information*, for example, about a patient's condition or the pros and cons of various treatment options.

- To *gather information* from a patient about their symptoms, their medical history or their preferred options for treatment.

- To *reassure* a patient, to empathise with a client or to alleviate anxiety for a service user.

- To *build rapport* and trust with patients and colleagues (and relatives, who are vital partners in a patient's recovery).

- To *explain* to a patient their diagnosis, a medical procedure or a hospital policy.

- To *persuade* a patient to do something such as to take their medication, to brush their teeth more often, to lose weight or to exercise more.

Why effective communication is vital

What Examples 1.1 and 1.2 demonstrate is the importance of effective communication, as opposed to just communication for its own sake. Professor Dianne Berry,[10] Dean of Postgraduate Research Studies at the University of Reading, says: 'We need to impart the right information, to the right people, in the right way, at the right time. Simply providing more information per se cannot be a goal in itself.' Professor Berry highlights important considerations. For communication to be effective, it needs to be relevant and accurate, targeted, timely and in the right format.

Being good at communicating will stand you in good stead in many aspects of your life, from relationships with friends and loved ones to your dealings with colleagues. But as people working in health and social care, you – perhaps more than others – must be effective communicators. Lives may depend on it. We've all heard stories about the wrong leg being amputated following a communications failure. Thankfully that kind of so-called 'never event' is rare (see Chapter 9 for more information on never events), but communications failures still occur, and even quite minor ones can have serious repercussions – for staff, as well as patients. A 2015 American study[11] stated:

> 'We may not typically think of communication as a clinical skill, but health care providers and patients are frequently exposed to the tragic consequences of inadequate communication of critical information … [This] Report investigates how specific weaknesses in communication impact patient safety. When information falls through the cracks, diagnoses are confounded, procedures are complicated, and subsequent care is compromised.'

Communications failures between colleagues can result in healthcare professionals giving the wrong medication, or patients taking the wrong medication – or too much of the right one. Poor communication at handover from ambulance to hospital, or at the end of a shift, consultation or counselling session, can result in real harm to patients because important information is not passed from one professional to another. The American report cited above found that:

> 'Communication difficulties are not isolated to providers lacking 'people skills' or patients with language or comprehension deficits. Nor is the problem exclusive to communication that is misspoken or misunderstood: errors often

---

10 Berry D (2007) *Health Communication: Theory and practice*. Maidenhead: Open University Press.

11 CRICO Strategies (2015) *Malpractice Risks in Communication Failures 2015 Annual Benchmarking Report*. Available at: https://www.rmf.harvard.edu/Malpractice-Data/Annual-Benchmark-Reports/1-Request-CBS-Report-PDFs (accessed February 2017).

occur because information is unrecorded, misdirected, never received, never retrieved, or ignored. Every mode and system by which patients and caregivers share health-related information is vulnerable to failure.'

You entered healthcare to care for patients, so the risk that poor communication could harm them is justification enough to spend time improving the way you communicate. But there are plenty of other positive reasons why effective communication should be high on your list of priorities. One powerful motivator for enhancing your communication skills is that to be a truly effective healthcare or social care professional, you must be a highly effective communicator. Establishing a good rapport with your patient or client is the basis for an effective therapeutic relationship. If the patient does not understand what you are saying, feels that you are not listening to them, or your poor communication skills lead them to question your professional competence, there will be no rapport, no trust and no confidence. Patients will suffer, and their recovery will be delayed.

Conversely, good communicators can ease clients' anxieties by answering their questions in a clear and helpful manner or giving them information in a form that makes sense for them, allowing informed decisions to be reached. Good communicators are also better at taking accurate and relevant patient histories and thus picking up on factors that could be crucial to treatment and recovery. It is now widely believed that good communication is fundamental to quality of care and healing: patients are less likely to remember the technological interventions than the communication and human interaction from clinicians. They judge the quality of care they have received by that marker.[12] In short, service users have more confidence in professionals who can communicate effectively, which in turn makes it more likely that treatment regimens are followed or advice taken.

Patients and their relatives should be seen as co-partners in care, alongside the healthcare professional. To achieve this, they need good quality information that they can understand, and they need to be actively involved in discussions and decision making. To make informed decisions about their treatment and care, patients need healthcare professionals who are expert communicators, able to help facilitate that decision-making by providing information in a meaningful form. 'Many doctors aspire to excellence in diagnosing disease. Far fewer, unfortunately, aspire to the same standards of excellence in diagnosing what patients want,' says a 2012 King's Fund paper.[13] It goes on to say that if the NHS tackles this shortcoming, one of the victories will be that 'patients, who can

---

12 Jackie Jones in her foreword to McEwen A and Kraszewski S (Eds) (2010) *Communication Skills for Adult Nurses*. Maidenhead: Open University Press.

13 Mulley A, Trimble C & Elwyn G (2012) *Patients' Preferences Matter: Stop the silent misdiagnosis*. King's Fund.

suffer just as much from a preference misdiagnosis as a medical misdiagnosis, will get the medicine they would choose were they well informed – that is, if they had better information about treatment options, outcomes, and evidence.' Establishing patient preferences relies upon effective communication. Much research has suggested that patients would opt for fewer interventions were they better informed.

Practitioners in senior roles have the responsibility of being a good role model to new recruits and those working below them in the hierarchy, making it essential that they demonstrate exemplary communication skills at all times. By communicating effectively and placing a high value on communication as a key skill, you set the tone and encourage others to follow your good example, thereby developing a culture of effective communication in your workplace, from which everyone will benefit.

The importance of communication is evidenced by the fact that healthcare regulators require those on their registers to have and to use effective communication skills in their dealings with clients and colleagues. If you are a registered health or social care practitioner, your registration and livelihood depends on effective communication.

■ **General Medical Council** (GMC) in its guidance[14] states that doctors must 'listen to patients' and give them 'the information they want or need in a way they can understand'. Communication is one of the four domains of practice standards for doctors.

■ **Nursing and Midwifery Council** (NMC) states[15] that practitioners must be able to communicate clearly; use terms that patients, colleagues and the public can understand; take reasonable steps to meet people's language and communication needs, providing assistance to those who need help to communicate their own or other people's needs; use a range of verbal and non-verbal communication methods; check people's understanding to avert misunderstanding; and be able to communicate clearly and effectively in English.

■ **General Dental Council** (GDC) demands that dentists must 'Communicate effectively with patients – listen to them, give them time to consider information and take their individual views and communication needs into

---

14 General Medical Council (2013) *Good Medical Practice*. Available at: http://www.gmc-uk.org/guidance/good_medical_practice.asp (accessed February 2017).

15 NMC Code (2015) *Professional Standards of Practice and Behaviour for Nurses and Midwives*. Available at: https://www.nmc.org.uk/globalassets/sitedocuments/nmc-publications/nmc-code.pdf (accessed February 2017).

account' and 'Give patients the information they need, in a way they can understand, so that they can make informed decisions'.[16]

- **Health and Care Professions Council** (HCPC) regulates a host of different UK health professions, including biomedical scientists, podiatrists, dieticians, occupational therapists, paramedics, physiotherapists, radiographers, and speech and language therapists. Its guidance for students[17] requires practitioners to 'take all reasonable steps to make sure that you can communicate appropriately and effectively with service users and carers'.

- **General Pharmaceutical Council** (GPhC) asks its registrants[18] to 'communicate effectively with patients and the public and take reasonable steps to meet their communication needs.'

Serious breaches of your regulator's professional or ethical code of practice could result in an appearance before a fitness to practise (FtP) hearing. Communications failures are a feature in many complaints to the healthcare regulators. In the GMC's first ever 'state of the nation' report,[19] they delved into their data to show how lack of effective communication with patients, and poor or non-existent sharing of information with colleagues, has led to a significant number of formal complaints about doctors. In 2010 the GMC listed communication failures as one of its top three FtP concerns. Recurring issues included failure to provide appropriate information to patients, failure to listen, failure to meet communication needs, failure to provide or share information, and poor communication with young people.

As a former NMC FtP panel chair, I can testify that poor communication skills (including poor record-keeping) led to practitioners receiving a caution or even being removed from the Register. The vast majority of healthcare staff take seriously their duty to service users, to their professional regulator, to colleagues and to their employer to be a good communicator, and are extremely unlikely to appear before an FtP panel. Nevertheless, pay attention to communication – not only for defensive reasons to do with protecting your professional registration, but for positive reasons too. Improved communication will benefit you by making

16 General Dental Council (2013) *Standards for the Dental Team 2013*. Available at: http://www.gdc-uk.org/Dentalprofessionals/Standards/Documents/Standards%20for%20the%20Dental%20Team.pdf (accessed February 2017).

17 HCPC (2016) *Guidance on Conduct and Ethics for Students*. Available at: http://www.hpc-uk.org/assets/documents/10002c16guidanceonconductandethicsforstudents.pdf (accessed February 2017).

18 GPhC (2010, reprinted 2012) *Standards of Conduct, Ethics and Performance*. Available at: https://www.pharmacyregulation.org/sites/default/files/standards_of_conduct_ethics_and_performance_july_2014.pdf (accessed February 2017).

19 General Medical Council (2011) *The State of Medical Education and Practice in the UK*. Available at: http://www.gmc-uk.org/publications/10586.asp (accessed February 2017).

your day-to-day work more rewarding. By enhancing your interpersonal skills through excellent communication, you will boost your self-confidence, professional standing and career prospects; increase job satisfaction; and help reduce workplace stress. Effective communicators find that patients and colleagues respond to them positively, creating a more affirmative, supportive working environment. But crucially, effective communication protects patients from potential harm arising from misunderstandings. All of the above are powerful positive reasons for striving to become an excellent communicator.

Reflection

All it takes is one charismatic communicator to set the tone for positive communication to become the norm in a workplace. Look around you to see if there is anyone whose communication style you would like to emulate. Learn from them. Watch how they deal with situations, and see how you can apply their techniques to improve the way that you communicate with others.

Even outside of work or study, effective communication can enrich your life, making for a happier, more harmonious household with stronger friendships and more fulfilling family relationships. It's a virtuous circle, because if you're happier out of work, you'll have fewer domestic troubles to preoccupy you and damage your ability to communicate when you are at work.

It is generally agreed that effective communication enhances the patient experience and the all-important therapeutic relationship; it reduces complaints and the costs associated with complaints handling; it improves patient health; it saves the NHS money; and it makes work more rewarding for practitioners. In this way, good communication benefits patients/service users, staff and organisations: everybody gains.

Attributes of a good communicator

Think about the attributes of an effective communicator and aim to embody them yourself. Good communicators are easy to talk to, skilled at putting patients and others at ease, and able to build rapport with a wide range of people. They display all or most of the following attributes. The good communicator:

- accurately assesses the needs of others, whether expressed through verbal or non-verbal indicators
- uses language that is appropriate for the audience

- listens actively and concentrates on what is being said

- asks open questions to gain information

- demonstrates they are listening by nodding, smiling, and in other ways, as appropriate

- displays open, encouraging and appropriate body language (facial expressions, eye contact and posture)

- responds appropriately to other people's verbal cues and body language

- thinks before responding

- checks that they have understood and have been understood

- seeks clarification where necessary

- corrects any misunderstandings

- reflects on their performance, and tries to learn from encounters and to improve their skills.

Poor communication

It is self-evident that if being a good communicator produces positive results for patients and staff, being a poor communicator produces suboptimal outcomes. A succession of bodies – from the Care Quality Commission in England to the Parliamentary and Health Service Ombudsman in England and the Scottish Public Services Ombudsman – record that poor communication lies at the heart of many complaints about healthcare organisations and individual practitioners. The Health Service Ombudsman says:[20]

> 'The NHS Constitution highlights the importance of good communication in order to build trust between healthcare providers and patients and their families. Despite this, poor communication is still one of the most common reasons for people to bring complaints about the NHS to the Ombudsman. Poor communication during care or treatment … can undermine successful clinical treatment, turning a patient's story of their experience with the NHS from one of success to one of frustration, anxiety and dissatisfaction. Good communication involves asking for feedback, listening to patients, and understanding their concerns and the outcome they are looking for. It is

---

20 Parliamentary and Health Service Ombudsman (2010-11) *Listening and Learning: The ombudsman's review of complaint handling by the NHS in England*. Available at: http://www. ombudsman.org.uk/__data/assets/pdf_file/0019/12286/Listening-and-Learning-Screen.pdf (accessed February 2017).

about keeping patients and their families informed and giving them clear, prompt, accurate, complete and empathetic explanations for decisions. Issues of confidentiality, insensitive or inappropriate language, use of jargon and a failure to take account of patients' own expertise in their condition feature frequently in complaints.'

Poor communication also wastes vast amounts of scarce NHS money, according to a report[21] for cancer charity Marie Curie by former top civil servant Andrew McDonald. Speaking only about England, he says:

'We do not know the full extent of waste generated through poor communications but this report argues that it is in excess of £1 billion. This waste is evident in poor adherence to medication regimes, repeat visits to clinics, disputes and, ultimately, litigation.'

Other research supports this view that poor communication is costly, in monetary terms and in terms of the human cost to patients.

The Care Quality Commission's 2011 inpatient survey recorded that 67% of patients said that they always received answers that they could understand from doctors (66% for nurses). The remainder said this occurred sometimes (27% for doctors, 29% for nurses) or never (6% for doctors, 5% for nurses). This is nowhere near good enough, because it means that around a third of patients are receiving answers that they do not understand some or all of the time. No healthcare professional would set out to confound a patient with complex and impenetrable answers, but that is sometimes the outcome.

Always be open to the possibility that poor communication may be of your making – perhaps you conveyed an over-complex message; were ambiguous; or simply failed to recognise that a patient was so preoccupied with pain or so worried about symptoms that they were unable to listen attentively and absorb the message (see Figure 1.2 on p.13). Regardless of good intentions, everyone will get it wrong sometimes. Take responsibility for trying to put things right when they do go awry. If you fail to identify and correct communications errors, and simply continue to communicate regardless of whether your words are being heard, understood or digested, you are effectively talking to yourself rather than engaging in meaningful dialogue. The sooner miscommunication is recognised and corrected, the more likely you will be to get a relationship back on track. (In the next chapter, consideration is given to physical, emotional and psychological

---

21 McDonald A for Marie Curie (2016) *A Long and Winding Road: Improving communication with patients in the NHS*. Available at: https://www.mariecurie.org.uk/globalassets/media/documents/policy/campaigns/the-long-and-winding-road.pdf (accessed February 2017).

barriers that can impede communication and there is an exploration of practical ways of overcoming them.)

Practitioners can perhaps be forgiven for well-intentioned but failed communications attempts: at least we tried, even if we did not succeed. It is much harder to understand the practitioner who makes no attempt at all, or who sees no need for communication.

True story

My husband Paul severed his thumb with a machete. The plastic surgeon took his medical history and reattached the detached digit. A week later, Paul visited the pharmacy to collect his repeat prescription hypertension medication, only to find that the plastic surgeon had instructed the GP to suspend it. It was two weeks before he was able to get it reinstated. In the meantime, Paul suffered from severe headaches, a direct result of being deprived of his usual medication. The surgeon did not communicate her decision to Paul, let alone discuss it, explain it or consult with him to understand his needs and wishes. This arrogant communication failure on her part led to two weeks of unnecessary discomfort for her patient.

Arrogance is not the only reason for lack of communication. The culture within healthcare can sometimes lead to staff unwittingly becoming unthinking and desensitised, seeing patients as a series of symptoms (or in need solely of tasks to be performed upon them) rather than as human beings with social and emotional needs. This leads to basic communications failures such as not introducing oneself, which can leave a patient feeling dehumanised. The 'hello my name is' campaign was created by Dr Kate Granger MBE, a registrar in elderly medicine who had terminal cancer and died in 2016. She started the campaign in 2013 after encountering NHS staff who failed to introduce themselves when providing care to her as an inpatient. Dr Granger asked NHS staff to pledge to introduce themselves to their patients. It is such an easy thing to do, yet it can have such a beneficial effect.

Dr Granger wrote on her blog:[22]

> 'As a healthcare professional you know so much about your patient. You know their name, their personal details, their health conditions, who they live with and much more. What do we as patients know about our healthcare professionals? The answer is often absolutely nothing, sometimes it seems not even their names. The balance of power is very one-sided in favour of the healthcare professional.'
> 'I have always been a strong believer in getting to know people's names as part

---

22 www.drkategranger.wordpress.com.

of building good working relationships with both patients and other colleagues. I think it is the first rung on the ladder to providing compassionate care, and often getting the simple things right, means the more complex things will follow more easily and naturally.'

As Dr Granger found, it sometimes requires an experience as a patient (or relative of a patient), for healthcare practitioners to be reminded of the importance of the small things that can be given little consideration by staff, but which are fundamental to the experience of patients. In an article for the *Journal of the American Medical Association*,[23] a doctor wrote of his experiences accompanying his elderly father to hospital: 'An unidentified young woman in a white coat stood sheepishly behind the surgeon. Never introduced or acknowledged, she also remained nameless.' It was the same when they met the anaesthetist, who also failed to ask 'any personal or social questions. His lack of interest in us as individuals was disheartening.' The author reflected on his medical training:

'My mentors imparted to me that little things, like shaking hands with each person in the room, asking their names … can develop trust and co-operation. Now I know it is true. Greeting a patient by name can bridge a huge gulf filled with fear and uncertainty. It is such a simple act to strengthen such an important relationship.'

Practitioners with poor communication skills

Think of someone you have encountered who is a poor communicator. They most likely sometimes make patients or colleagues feel awkward, nervous, ill at ease, unwelcome or even afraid. Such a person may at times appear distracted, in a hurry, bored or uninterested in what is being said. They may well reply in a dismissive or patronising fashion or respond in a judgemental way. There is a chance that they are discourteous, such as ignoring the patient/client and speaking to a colleague or taking a phone call. Their behaviour is likely to be a combination of several of the following:

- defensive, aggressive or rude
- loud and pushy, or excessively quiet and withdrawn
- does not listen, or listens but fails to demonstrate active listening
- mumbles, mutters or does not speak clearly
- speaks in a wordy way rather than being succinct

23 Bruder Stapleton F (2000) My name is Jack. *Journal of the American Medical Association*, **284** (16) 2027.

- curt, lacking social niceties and 'small talk'

- uses jargon that the listener is unlikely to understand

- interrupts frequently or finishes others' sentences

- uses inappropriate body language and other non-verbal signals and gestures, such as standing too close (or too far away), folding their arms or frowning

- does not make appropriate eye contact – too much (making the other person feel under scrutiny and uncomfortable) or not enough

- fails to notice or to respond to other people's non-verbal cues, or responds inappropriately

- does not provide the patient with information, or even recognise the need for this

- asks closed or leading questions and does not encourage two-way conversation.

It may be tempting to dismiss poor communicators as uncaring individuals, but that would be incorrect. Much suboptimal communication stems from the well-intentioned actions of people who are simply lacking in knowledge and confidence about how to communicate effectively. People learn by emulating others, so if there are poor communicators in your team, you may pick up some of their poor practice. Always keep a check on your own style, and if appropriate, give constructive feedback to others.

True story

While in hospital, a nurse came to my bed and told me that she needed to take my blood pressure. She did so, and duly wrote the results in my notes. Job done – except that she failed to tell me what the reading was, whether it was normal, or why it was necessary. In fact, she said nothing at all about it. It didn't occur to her that I might be relieved to hear her say: 'Good news. Your blood pressure has come down and is now completely normal.' She regarded this as a task to be completed rather than an opportunity to reassure a worried patient.

Ethical communication

Medical ethics is a familiar concept to those working in healthcare; ethical healthcare communication less so. Communication can be used for good and bad – just think about political propaganda and how it has been employed to manipulate opinion and influence thinking. Communications techniques can be deployed in a patient-centric way to empower clients and actively involve them in decision-making about their care. Equally, they can be used inappropriately to exert influence and to persuade in a way that takes control away from patients.

- *Ethical communication* involves presenting healthcare information in a neutral, honest and balanced way to a patient, so that they can weigh up the pros and cons and reach an informed decision on next steps. It involves admitting when you do not know the answer or when there is conflicting evidence.

- *Unethical communication* involves presenting information in a biased, manipulated or misleading way – such as unduly stressing highly unlikely side effects – to persuade, influence or coax the patient into taking the option that you want them to take. It can involve failure to admit to a lack of knowledge, and omitting to present information that does not support your view.

Unethical communication can sometimes occur as a result of the best intentions, but it remains unethical. The practitioner might genuinely believe that they know what is in the patient's best interests, or think that the patient is making a serious error in their choice of treatment (or non-treatment). That does not give the healthcare practitioner the right to withhold information or present biased or false information. Without full, unbiased information, how can a patient give informed consent?

Identifying and understanding strengths and weaknesses

So, are you a poor communicator or a good one? Most of us try to be effective communicators, but sometimes we make mistakes. Our communication style may vary according to the situation. We could be great at talking to our friends, but not so good at communicating with service users. Or perhaps we're generally good with patients, but we find it really hard to break bad news. Maybe we're OK most of the time, but face difficulties when tired or stressed.

Reflection

Identify situations where you communicate well, and others where you need to try harder. What practical things can you do to correct any weaknesses? (Revisit this reflective exercise once you've completed the book and have a few more practical ideas for improving your communication style.)

Spend time reflecting on how you communicate. Think about the kind of communication you find easy, and the things, people or situations you find hard. Try to understand yourself a little better. Become conscious of your communication style and analyse your strengths and weaknesses. Observe your colleagues too. Over the next week or so, try to be aware of how you communicate. Jot down any observations in a communications diary, and review the diary once you have completed the book. Keep a note of the outcomes of the reflective exercises too.

Communication style: self-awareness test

Work through the following questions. Be totally honest with yourself when answering.

Do you find it harder to communicate certain information at work (for example, to ask about 'difficult' or sensitive things such as sexual health)?

....

....

....

What things do you find hard to communicate at work and why?

....

....

....

....

Do you find it easy to communicate certain information (for example, to ask about or to provide simple factual information)?

....

....

....

What sorts of things do you find easy and why?

....

....

....

....

Do you find it harder to communicate with some groups, such as children or people with a learning disability?

....

....

....

Which groups do you find harder to communicate with?

....

....

....

Why might this be?

....

....

....

Do you find it easier to communicate with certain groups (such as people who are similar to you or your friends)?

....

....

....

Which groups do you find it easier to communicate with?

....

....

....

Why might this be?

....

....

....

At work, in what sorts of situations do you find it hard to communicate and why (for example, when people are angry or upset)?

....

....

....

What do you actively do to make patients (and relatives) feel heard/listened to?

....

....

....

Do you have a tendency to interrupt, finish sentences for others or talk too much?

....

....

....

If yes, in what kinds of situations?

....

....

....

Do you make assumptions about certain groups and amend your usual communication as a result?

....

....

....

If you answered yes, which groups?

....

....

....

Are your assumptions correct? How do you know? (Some assumptions can be positive and can lead to improved communication – such as simplifying what you say when talking to young children – but others can be negative, even discriminatory, and can impede communication.)

....

....

....

Has a particular style of communication developed in your workplace and, if so, what style and what is its impact? (In some workplaces, communication can become rushed, and this can leave people feeling that they are not listened to.)

....

....

....

Reflection

Think about how you and your colleagues communicate with patients and each other. Reflect on whether any improvements can and should be made to habits or patterns of communication that have become the norm in your surgery/ward/clinic/workplace. Don't be afraid to ask a friend or a trusted colleague about how you are perceived when you are in dialogue, and how you perform in different settings.

Reflect on the answers that you gave above. Return to the test in a month or so and consider whether you wish to revise any of the answers that you gave. Draw up an action plan to tackle any weaknesses and record it in your communications diary. Be specific about what you plan to do and when. Although the emphasis is inevitably on areas for improvement, remember to value your strengths too, and to build upon them.

Chapter 2: Barriers to effective communication

Communication never takes place in a vacuum: there is always a context. The patient might be stressed, anxious, eager to get home, or in severe pain, you might be tired, rushed, or worrying about a domestic matter. All of these factors can hamper communication. This chapter examines some of the barriers to communication – such as noise, lack of privacy, fear and pain – and suggests practical ways of overcoming them in order to aid effective communication.

Time and place are important contextual factors for successful communication. Practitioners with competing, sometimes urgent, pressures on their time may give insufficient attention to creating the right atmosphere (place) to transmit their message. We live in a pressured world where few practitioners complain of having too little to do. Lack of time is a common complaint, and it is self-evident that rushed communication will never be as good as a more leisurely interaction. When time is a luxury in short supply, you need to find ways to create quality communication. The deeper and more significant the conversation, the more time it will require – for preparation, as well as for the conversation itself.

For those working in hospitals, visiting time can provide a good opportunity to communicate with the patient and, where appropriate, to involve family or friends (obviously the patient's wishes regarding confidentiality must be taken into account). Even when there is no news to impart, frequent communication is important because it helps to develop the relationship and prepares the ground for more difficult conversations that may have to take place. This need not be time consuming: a smile, a hello, a wave or a sentence or two of small talk may suffice to sustain the relationship.

The inevitable competing demands that typically you find yourself juggling at work can divert attention and make you less attentive. As a result, you may fail to identify your patient's verbal and non-verbal signals. Sometimes it is entirely appropriate that you attend to an important task – such as relieving another patient's pain – but a simple 'I'll be with you just as soon as I've given Mrs Smith her painkillers' may be sufficient a communication to reassure a patient that they are on your radar.

Privacy

Failure to take account of the physical context in which communication occurs may result in problems, even when sufficient time is set aside to talk with a client. Few of us can fully control the environment in which we work, but it's important to be aware of the potential problems that our surroundings can create so that we can take this into consideration.

Patients are likely to be reticent about providing private or personal information if they are being asked their medical history in a quiet ward where other patients can hear the interaction clearly; at a busy reception desk; or in a cubicle with just a curtain for privacy. They may even give false answers. Just think about how you'd feel answering personal questions, or even just giving your weight, in full earshot of complete strangers, or worse, in front of neighbours or acquaintances at the local pharmacy or GP surgery.

True story

I visited my local chemist and requested to speak to the pharmacist. She came to the counter and asked, in front of everyone in the waiting queue, what I needed help with. It was a simple enquiry about Vitamin B12 supplements, but what if I'd wanted the morning-after pill, advice on constipation, or piles, or condoms? I might well have felt embarrassment. Consider how customers or clients may feel speaking to you in your working environment, and look at whether the physical layout or other arrangements may be improved to aid privacy where necessary and possible.

Dos and don'ts

- Do create the necessary privacy if you plan to ask about anything sensitive.

- Don't ask sensitive questions in busy areas. Take the patient to a quieter area or into a side room away from others, or ask others to step outside the room while you have the conversation.

- Do explore other ways of getting the information you need, such as asking the patient to complete a written form that gathers the pertinent facts (though don't forget that some patients may struggle with reading and writing).

Background noise

It's easy to become so familiar with your surroundings that you can no longer see the communication barriers that your workplace poses. Many practitioners thrive on the buzz of a busy clinic or day care centre, yet the inevitable background noise that is part of the comings and goings – the ringing phones, the ever-opening-and-closing doors, the noisy air conditioning – can compete with your message, especially (but not only) for patients with impaired hearing. It is not uncommon for people with a hearing impairment to try to disguise it by nodding and 'appearing' to hear. Be alert to that possibility. (Read more about the needs of people with a hearing impairment in Chapter 5.)

Dos and don'ts

- Do be aware of noise when speaking with service users and their families, as it may be a significant barrier to their ability to hear what you say – even if they are not hearing impaired.

- Don't forget that many people have a hearing impairment. Some clients might only partially hear what you say, which could lead to misunderstanding.

- Do turn the radio off, try to find a quiet corner, or step inside an office or side room if possible.

Too many stimuli

Busy areas full of distractions may create problems for patients who find it difficult to concentrate, particularly those with dementia and other cognitive impairments. It can be hard to focus when there's hustle and bustle all around. Activity and visual stimuli can interfere with the delivery of your message. (Read more about the needs of people with a cognitive impairment in Chapter 5.)

Dos and don'ts

- Do try to improve the conditions if you absolutely must speak to someone in a busy reception area or in a day room with a TV on in the corner. Your message will have to compete with everything else that is going on there. Reduce the volume/switch off the TV/radio, or preferably move to a quieter location.

■ Don't automatically have a conversation in the place where you or your client happen to be. Consider environment and, where possible, select the right surroundings in which to communicate important messages.

■ Do choose a time when things are less busy and there's less going on that may compete with your message.

■ Don't choose a slot when there's other competing planned activity (such as medicine rounds or meal times) that might interrupt your discussion.

Seating arrangements

Consider seating arrangements. Sitting behind a big desk creates a physical and psychological barrier between you and your patient (or colleague), which is likely to hinder effective communication by making the other person feel small, unimportant, insignificant or nervous. Careful consideration of the arrangement of any room in which patients are seen is vital if you wish to build a mutually respectful therapeutic relationship. Sitting at the same height as others will not in itself send out an egalitarian statement, but standing or sitting at a greater height than others certainly suggests a superior/inferior relationship that will not be conducive to effective communication.

Dos and don'ts

■ Do sit rather than stand when speaking with a patient in bed, sitting or using a wheelchair. Not only is it respectful to get down to their height; it makes it easier for the patient to hear you (and for you to hear them) and it conveys to them that both they and the conversation are important to you.

■ Don't let the physical layout of a room create barriers. Where a room can be arranged so that the desk/table does not appear as a barrier, do so. If you must sit at a desk, see if the seating can be arranged so that the service user sits at a right angle to you rather than opposite. This is a less confrontational, more intimate seating arrangement.

■ Do position yourself where the patient can see your face and facial expressions clearly, if they cannot move their head, or their eyes, or need to lipread.

Reflection

Take a high chair or a tall stool and ask a colleague to sit in it. You can take up position on a low seat. Have a conversation with your colleague and think about how it feels to be so much physically lower than the other person. For an even more lowly experience, place a big desk between the two of you. Reflect on what it must be like for patients when seating is so arranged. What message does such an arrangement communicate?

Table 2.1 suggests practical ways to ensure the best circumstances for effective communication. Think about your own working environment, any circumstances that may create suboptimal communication, and any actions you can take to remedy the situation.

Table 2.1: Effects of context on communication and practical remedies

Circumstance	Effect	Action
Competing demands on practitioner's time.	■ Rushed or poorly prepared communication. ■ Little or no time for eliciting questions from clients or answering them. ■ Practitioner may appear distracted, uninterested or uncaring.	■ Wherever possible, choose a less rushed time to initiate communication, although urgent situations may preclude this. ■ Acknowledge that you are busy, and apologise for having to rush. ■ If appropriate, agree a time when you will return to address any questions or concerns, or ensure that a colleague does so.

Competing noise from other patients, staff, visitors or equipment.	■ You may have to raise your voice, risking the possibility that this will make you appear angry, impatient or uncaring. ■ Your range of verbal subtlety will be reduced in these circumstances.	■ Choose a quiet room or a quieter time to have important conversations. ■ Reduce noise by requesting silence; by closing doors/windows; by waiting until the cleaner has switched the vacuum off.
Service user's sensory impairment.	■ They may unable to hear your message, or see your face or 'read' your body language.	■ Ensure that physical aids are available and are working – such as checking that a hearing aid is in place, that spectacles are worn, or that the lighting is good.
Patient's examination or treatment at out-patient clinic such as breast, colposcopy, colo-rectal or genitourinary clinic.	■ Patient's fear and anxiety about cancer may impair their ability to listen or to retain information.	■ Address patient's concerns by providing facts, explanations and, where appropriate, reassurance. ■ Consider giving written information that can be taken home and read later – or in advance of the consultation/treatment.

Addressing time and space issues to reflect the importance and degree of urgency of the conversation is vital, but even then, and regardless of how fluent or articulate a practitioner you are, there is no guarantee that every communication with every service user will be successful. For a communication to be effective, the message received must be the same as the intended message (see Figure 1.1, Chapter 1). Even clear, unambiguous messages can become distorted in transmission, thus preventing them from being received in their intended form. The following are some of the other factors that can interfere with the receipt of messages or influence how they are interpreted or whether they are understood.

Pain

Do you have to deal with patients who are in pain? Even mild pain or discomfort can reduce a patient's ability to pay due attention. It can be hard to get your message across when a casualty is lying on the roadside with four cracked ribs, or on a hospital trolley contending with the distractions of a throbbing head, smarting eyes, aching legs and a sore back. What can you do in such situations to help ensure that your message is received?

Dos and don'ts

- Do offer analgesia if appropriate (and within your scope of practice) and acknowledge their pain and discomfort: 'I know that you're in a great deal of pain, but it's important that I discuss with you …'

- Don't overlook the benefits of 'small talk' as an important phase in establishing a rapport with a patient, but don't let it dominate and divert attention from the information that you really need to impart.

- Do consider whether this is the best time to impart your message. Is the patient's pain likely to ease soon and can your message wait until then?

- Don't forget that the patient may be unable to give you their full attention. Ask if there is anything they would like repeated.

- Do think about whether your message could be broken into bite-size pieces so there is less to digest in one go: 'I will explain about your medication now, and I'll come back after lunch to tell you about how physiotherapy may help.'

Fatigue

Sometimes you may have to speak to people who are tired or drowsy: perhaps the patient's condition has kept them awake all night; or they're coming round from an anaesthetic; have consumed a large amount of alcohol or taken illegal drugs; or a client's medication is making them a bit sleepy. It can be difficult communicating with people who are not fully alert and receptive to your message, but there are things you can do to make it easier.

Dos and don'ts

- Do acknowledge their fatigue: 'I know that you've had a bad night and you're tired now, but …' Showing empathy can help build a rapport and make a patient more receptive to you.

- Don't forget to stress the importance of your message, so that they know that their attention is required: 'It's really important that you listen to this because …'

- Do consider whether this is the best time to impart your message. Is their fatigue likely to lessen, and can your message wait until then? Can you deliver part of the message now and the rest later, so there is less to take in at once?

- Don't forget to check for understanding and consider repeating the message: 'It can be difficult to take everything in when you're tired, so I just wanted to check that you're clear about …' If the communication is very important, ask the patient to replay it back to you, as this aids retention of information and serves as a useful check to you that they've understood.

Fear and anxiety

The Care Quality Commission's *2015 Inpatient Survey: Statistical release*[24] recorded that 71 percent of patients said that they always received answers that they could understand from doctors and nurses when asking an important question. The figure fell to just 54 percent for people with a learning disability and 52 percent for those with a mental health condition, when asking a doctor a question (the figure for nurses was slightly better). These figures show a steady improvement over previous years but remain nowhere near good enough, because almost a third of patients are receiving answers that they do not understand some or all of the time. No healthcare professional would set out to confound a patient with complex and impenetrable answers, but that is sometimes the outcome.

Dos and don'ts

- Do calm fears first, then make your point: 'Try to relax. The ambulance is on its way. Can you show me where it hurts?'; 'It's understandable that you're nervous, but there's no need. Lots of people safely go through this procedure every week …'

- Don't ignore body language (more on that in Chapter 3). If you smile or in some other way look approachable, clients will feel more inclined to listen to you and more able to discuss their worries or concerns.

- Do make the environment less clinical if possible, so that patients or clients feel less anxious or intimidated. Simple and affordable measures such as a

---

24 Care Quality Commission (2016) *2015 Inpatient Survey: Statistical release*. Available at: http://www.cqc.org.uk/sites/default/files/20150822_ip15_statistical_release_corrected.pdf (accessed February 2017).

calming colour on the walls, a few pictures, or a pot plant can all reduce stress. If you are not a budget-holder for such items, discuss it with someone who is.

Deference and awe

It is generally agreed that the days of widespread and automatic deference for clinicians is behind us, but some patients – anecdotally it seems to be primarily the older generation, though not always – retain great respect for and deference towards healthcare professionals, particularly practitioners at the upper end of the hierarchy. Such patients may be reluctant, or even unwilling, to ask questions, ask for clarification or ask for information to be repeated. They may fear that their questions are too simple or will make them appear stupid. Clients may worry about 'wasting a busy professional's time with daft questions'. There are many ways to counter this and to encourage people to engage with you.

Dos and don'ts

- Do encourage questions, perhaps even suggesting that you expect them. Ask directly whether the client has questions, and use prompts and open questions: 'You're bound to have questions. What can I answer for you?'; 'What else can I tell you about the operation?'; or 'What would you like to know about the next steps?'

- Don't neglect to emphasise that there's no such thing as a silly question.

- Do anticipate and address likely anxieties: 'Will I be in pain?'; 'Will I get better?'; 'Will I have to change how I live my life?'; 'Will I be able to have sex again?'; or even 'Will I die?'

- Don't forget to reinforce the fact that their health or welfare is your job: tell service users that you're paid to help them, and they need never worry about taking up your time if they are worried or uncertain.

Embarrassment

Would you feel comfortable talking about your sex life, difficult family circumstances, fears, addictions or bowel problems with a complete stranger, or having to undress in front of them? Probably not. Nor do most patients. Their embarrassment, or indeed a practitioner's embarrassment, can result in an awkward and uncomfortable encounter that interferes with effective communication. Anticipating and acting to minimise embarrassment, combined with straightforward, open communication, can ease the situation for all.

Be clear, direct and explicit with patients. Don't say 'Please undress,' as this can leave patients worried and unsure about what that means. Should they take everything off, or just outer clothing? Pants on or off? You know what's expected for the examination, but they may not. A more specific instruction such as 'Please remove your trousers and pants, but keep your T-shirt on' is clear and unambiguous. Such directions can ease stress and embarrassment when delivered with matter-of-fact confidence. However, a lack of confidence will be detected by a patient and may add to the awkwardness of the situation for both of you.

Service users may not always know what is acceptable or 'normal'. Patients may be unsure about what words are appropriate for referring to various parts of the anatomy or bodily functions. Clients may worry about shocking or embarrassing you. It is natural for people to fear having to undress or to undergo an intimate examination. Patients may feel mortified about having an 'accident' and having someone clean up their soiled clothes or bedding. Such embarrassment can create a barrier and hamper communication. Think about ways of helping ease such embarrassing situations, enabling everyone to concentrate on communicating rather than worrying. Table 2.2 suggests practical ways to help deal with patients' embarrassment.

Table 2.2: Practical ways to manage embarrassment and ease communication

Circumstance	Effect	Action
Flatulence, vomiting and other bodily excretions.	■ Acute embarrassment and possible revulsion by patient. ■ Inhibition that may deter patient from seeking help from those caring for them. ■ Physical and emotional discomfort, which may hamper communication.	■ Anticipate what circumstances may occur and discuss these with the patient before they happen. ■ If possible, provide the physical means to minimise concern and embarrassment, such as sanitary towels or clean underwear. ■ Emphasise that it is the patient's condition, not the patient, that is responsible for this. ■ Deal with the situation quickly, matter-of-factly and without fuss.

Intimate examination.	■ Patient may feel exposed (physically and psychologically), vulnerable and unhappy. ■ Embarrassment may prevent them from listening or asking questions.	■ Explain why the examination is necessary and provide an opportunity to ask questions. ■ Communicate what the examination will involve, in a way the patient can understand, so that they have a clear idea of what to expect. ■ Protect patients' dignity by ensuring maximum privacy (curtains fully drawn, modesty blanket, gowns that fit and fasten) – and allowing them privacy to undress/dress. ■ Do not make unnecessary personal comments. ■ Allow patients time to dress and recompose before discussing examination findings with them. ■ Offer patients a chaperone such as another healthcare professional, even if you are the same gender as the patient. Reschedule the examination (if delay has no adverse effect on the patient's health) if a suitable chaperone is not immediately available.

Client needs to discuss intimate problem but is unsure what vocabulary to use to refer to body parts or functions.	■ Client may be quiet or reserved, avert eyes, withhold key information, provide false answers, or reveal only those parts that they feel comfortable talking about.	■ Set the tone by using the vocabulary that the client may be searching for. ■ A useful technique is to introduce words such as 'bowel movements' or 'penis' into your questions, if you think they may be at a loss as to what terminology to use. Words such as 'stool', which have a different everyday meaning, may cause confusion.

Embarrassment may stem from things that surprise you: a patient may be embarrassed by the untidiness of their house or flat when the doctor, community health practitioner or paramedic calls, to such a degree that they are not paying attention to what you are saying.

Dos and don'ts

■ Do smile to ease the tension (but beware inappropriate smiles – such as when giving bad news or discussing intimate matters). Use positive, open body language.

■ Don't miss signs of embarrassment: not just the obvious ones, such as blushing, but laughter, joking, fidgeting and other behaviours aimed at masking it.

■ Do offer reassurance if a client apologises for the state of their accommodation: 'Please don't worry. Let's just concentrate on you.'

■ Don't sound disapproving or judgemental when asking about sensitive issues. Be careful how you phrase questions. 'You don't drink more than ten glasses of wine a week, do you?' is likely to make the client feel that the 'right' or desired answer is 'no'. Increase the chances of eliciting a more truthful answer with a neutral, open question: 'How many glasses of wine do you drink in a typical week?'

> **Reflection**
>
> Think about the last time you were really embarrassed. How did you feel? What might have made you feel better in that situation? How might you apply that learning to your encounters with clients?

Jargon

Most professions have their own jargon. It can be an important aid in professional-to-professional communication between those in the same field, but be cautious about using technical jargon and clinical acronyms with a patient. They may not know what you are talking about and could be reluctant to ask for a plain English translation.[25] It is easy to slip into jargon without realising it, so make a conscious effort to avoid it. A Royal College of General Practitioners' report[26] cited the example of a patient who was told that their cancer diagnosis was 'positive'. They took this to be good (i.e. 'positive') news, when the reverse was the case.

Dos and don'ts

- Do beware of ambiguity. Words that may have one meaning for a practitioner may have another in common parlance, such as 'acute' or 'stool'.

- Don't use vocabulary that is inappropriate for the audience. Grown-up language will probably not be understood by a young child,[27] so ensure that communication is age-appropriate when speaking with children and young people (more on that in Chapter 5). Do not use belittling, childish, or over-familiar expressions with older people. Complex sentence structures, slang (very informal words and expressions) or too fast a pace used when speaking to someone who is not fluent in English will leave your listener with a puzzled look.

- Do explain what you mean if you really need to use jargon. It's best to keep things simple: say kidney, not 'renal'; heart, not 'cardio'.

---

25 See www.plainenglish.co.uk for real examples of healthcare jargon.

26 Royal College of General Practitioners (2014) *Health Literacy: Report from an RCGP-Led Health Literacy Workshop*. Available at: http://www.rcgp.org.uk/clinical-and-research/clinical-resources/health-literacy-report.aspx (accessed February 2017).

27 The Patient Information Forum's (2010) *Guide to Producing Health Information for Children and Young People* says that the complexity of children's thinking increases with age, and their views about health and illness vary with their level of cognitive development. As a result, practitioners need to present information in different ways, depending on the different stages of a young person's development.

- Don't say: 'There's an 80% chance that …' The mention of percentages, even simple ones, can be confusing. It may be better to say that 'Eight out of ten people …' This humanises the statistic and makes it less mathematical.

- Do consider using easy-to-relate-to analogies when explaining things, such as 'Your bowel is a bit like a garden hose.'

Language

If someone is not a native English speaker, and they are not proficient in the language, this will pose a very real communication barrier. Interpreting and translation services such as Languageline are available. For more detailed information and advice on communicating with patients whose first language is not English, see Chapter 5.

Reflection

Think about recent encounters with service users. What communications barriers have you come across? How can you amend your communication style to take account of these factors so that your message is not missed, diluted or distorted?

Values and beliefs

Everyone makes assumptions based on their social or cultural beliefs, values and traditions, biases and prejudices. Practitioners should be aware of their own cultural norms and be careful not to allow them to interfere with communication or hamper the therapeutic relationship. At the same time, it helps to be alert to other people's values and beliefs. Differences can lead practitioner, or patient, to misinterpret what is said, to reinterpret it, or to simply ignore it.

For example, a patient might genuinely believe that female staff must be junior, or that a man cannot be a midwife. This can result in the patient giving insufficient attention to advice offered by a female practitioner. Think about how you can address situations like this. Consider explaining your role at the outset: 'Hello, I am the doctor who will be examining you today.' Or, 'I am the social worker who will be handling your case.'

A practitioner might believe that a patient in a same-sex relationship will not have children, that an Asian client will not speak good English, or that someone

with a learning disability or an older person will not be in an active sexual relationship. Incorrect assumptions can cause offence and damage the therapeutic relationship. Even innocently intended enquiries may cause offence. Asking someone's 'Christian name' may be culturally insensitive for non-Christians, for example. Asking a man what his 'wife' thinks is inappropriate, unless you know that he has one – people may be single or in same-sex relationships. Stick to neutral words like 'partner'. Try to identify your own assumptions, prejudices and values. Reflect on how they could impact at work. What can you do to ensure that there is no negative impact? Remember that we are not all the same. Not everyone thinks like you or believes what you believe. Respect differences.

True story

Jenny[28] became unwell in the park, and a passer-by dialled 999 and waited for the ambulance to arrive. He showed the paramedics Jenny's medic alert bracelet, but they didn't look at it and assessed her as having a panic attack. Jenny said, 'By dismissing my symptoms as just a panic attack, I was made to feel like I was wasting their time. They didn't seem to want to do even basic observations.'

On arrival at A&E, paramedics reported her 'panic attack', and Jenny was left in the waiting area. She says, 'The triage nurse talked to me with disdain, again making me feel like I was a time-waster. She asked me why I felt that this was an emergency, and didn't seem interested in the fact that I hadn't called the ambulance, nor that I was genuinely ill. I felt that I had been stereotyped. I've had a lot of experience with mental health services over the years and I felt that the healthcare staff were of the view that I was a waste of their precious resources.

'Finally I saw a doctor. He listened to me and made me feel that he genuinely cared that I was feeling unwell. He arranged for some tests. Why the different attitude? He'd accessed my hospital records and was aware of the information held on my medic alert bracelet, which explained that I have a brain tumour and am awaiting treatment.'

Had the ambulance crew not jumped to the wrong conclusion about Jenny, they would have seen that she was ill. Had they taken notice of her bracelet, they would have known why she was ill, and could have communicated this to the receiving staff at the hospital. Jenny could have received treatment faster and more compassionately.

---

28 Not her real name.

She told me, 'It would seem that being prejudged by the ambulance crew led to hostility from A&E staff, which was only resolved when the doctor accessed my clinical information. I feel this is a disgusting way to approach patients, and also highly judgemental. Thankfully, on this occasion no harm was caused. My consultants have told me that should I feel uncharacteristically unwell I ought to dial 999. I will absolutely hesitate to do so after this experience. Feeling unwell and being treated like this is remarkably upsetting, never mind having to cope with the pain and treatment that comes with a brain tumour.'

- Why do you think the paramedics treated Jenny in this way?
- Do you think that their actions were influenced by value judgements that they reached about Jenny based on non-clinical factors? If so, what factors might they have taken into account?
- What is the danger in jumping to conclusions based on non-clinical factors?
- What message has Jenny taken away with her following that encounter?

After that negative healthcare experience, Jenny wrote about what happened to her on the Patient Opinion website.[29] The ambulance service in question engaged with Jenny to address her concerns, learn from her experience, and take action to prevent any reoccurrence.

Reflection

Think about a situation where you have reached a conclusion about someone that later proved to be wrong. What made you jump to the wrong conclusion? How did you feel when you realised that you had got it wrong? Was any damage caused? Remember that false assumptions need not be negative. Have you been on the receiving end of prejudice? How did it make you feel?

---

29 Patient Opinion (www.patientopinion.org.uk) believes that patients' feedback, good or bad, is essential to improving UK health services. It passes patients' stories to those in the health services who can make a difference. Jenny's story was given to the Scottish Ambulance Service (SAS), who contacted Jenny to discuss her experiences. Feedback was provided to the paramedics in question, and now Jenny is helping the SAS as a patient representative on the project board for the development of their mental health care pathway.

Information overload

It is not uncommon for patients to complain that they have not been given enough information, but be aware that it's also possible to communicate too much, which can create problems in itself. Most of us find it difficult to take in a lot of information in one go and glaze over if we are bombarded with facts and figures, statistics, options and alternatives. It's all just too much. This is particularly true for patients who are upset, distressed, anxious, tired, in shock or in pain. It also applies to patients who lack capacity. But we can all find it difficult to take in lengthy information or complex messages. When you have to impart a lot of information:

■ Set out clearly what information you are providing and why.

■ Devote more time to what is most important – and flag up when a particular piece of information is particularly important: 'You need to pay particular attention to this because it's really important …'

■ If you know in advance that you will have a lot of information to impart, consider offering the client the option of involving a relative or friend in the conversation, two pairs of ears being better than one. (The patient may not wish others to know their business. Respect their wishes on confidentiality and disclosure.)

■ Suggest that the client takes notes if they wish.

■ With the consent of the patient, some practitioners make a recording[30] of their session together and give the client a copy so they can listen to it again later.

■ Consider whether it would be appropriate for a client to record part of the consultation on their mobile phone, so that they can replay it later or share it with a partner who was unable to accompany them.

Dos and don'ts

■ Do keep to the pertinent information.

■ Don't forget that written information can supplement or reinforce what is said. It can be read at a later time when the client may be more able to digest it.

■ Do arrange another meeting if necessary, either to go over details again or to provide further information.

■ Don't forget to find out if there is anything more that the patient wants to know.

---

30 Consult your own regulatory body for a copy of their guidance on recording patients.

Practitioner barriers

So far, we have focused on barriers that stand between patients and their ability to give and receive information. Here we look at the barriers that impede healthcare practitioners' effective communication with patients and colleagues.

Practitioner appearance and attitude are important ingredients of effective communication. Tiredness, an unprofessional appearance, or personal habits such as smoking, bad breath, body odour or poor hand hygiene all convey a negative message and reduce a practitioner's credibility among colleagues and patients. They may also be in breach of your employer's hand-hygiene or dress-code policies. Sufficient sleep, a healthy diet, good personal hygiene and high energy levels make communication more effective. They put up an invisible sign to the patient saying, 'You can have confidence in me. I'm a professional and I am in control of my life. I can help you to retain control when you are ill.' (You can read more about unintentional communication in the next chapter.)

Some overweight practitioners report that they feel that their healthy lifestyle messages have less credibility, as it is visible to patients that they have been unable to heed them. An article in the *Daily Mail*[31] supports the view that patients may not trust the advice of an obese doctor: 'It's ridiculous that any doctor with a belly overhanging their trousers should think they are fit to dish out medical advice, frankly,' TV presenter Steve Miller told the newspaper. The more distinguished *British Medical Journal*[32] reported, 'England's chief medical officer, Sally Davies, said that she was "perpetually surprised" at how many NHS staff were overweight. "How are they to have the impact on patients if they are not thinking about it for themselves?" she asked.'

An American study[33] of 500 primary care doctors found that overweight doctors were significantly less likely to discuss weight loss with overweight patients. Doctors with normal body mass index (BMI) reported greater confidence in their ability to provide diet and exercise advice, and perceived their weight-loss advice as trustworthy when compared to overweight or obese doctors. Whether doctors or patients should feel this way, the fact is that some do, and it can have a negative impact on some practitioners' ability to offer credible and persuasive advice on weight loss and healthy lifestyles. If you are overweight and need to communicate

---

31 Davies M (2015) Fat doctors 'should be struck off for setting a bad example to their obese patients', weight-loss expert tells NHS chief. *Mail Online* **6** July.

32 McCartney M (2014) Fat doctors are patients too. *BMJ* **349**. Available at: http://www.bmj.com/content/349/bmj.g6464 (accessed February 2017).

33 Bleich SN, Bandara S, Bennett WL, Cooper LA & Gudzune KA (2014) Impact of non-physician health professionals' BMI on obesity care and beliefs. *Obesity* **22** 2476–2480.

healthy-eating advice to others, reflect on how you can do so with confidence and authority, ensuring that your patients get the best advice from you.

Nervousness

Students and recently qualified practitioners will recall how nervous they were when having to speak to a patient alone for the first time. Nervousness is natural, but it must be controlled if its potentially negative impact is to be averted. Nervous people often forget to maintain eye contact; they may blush, stutter or frown; they may not remember to smile appropriately or to look sympathetic. Excessive nervousness can destroy your confidence in yourself and patients' confidence in you, so it needs to be addressed. While it is natural to be nervous, it is important to observe the following:

- Take steps to keep calm, such as deep breathing before entering a consulting room.

- Remember to pay attention to body language.

- Mentally rehearse your opening words so that they are fluent and put the patient at ease from the outset.

- If appropriate, tell the client that this is your first consultation and that you are a little nervous.

It is not only student practitioners who feel nervous. Locums, new staff and people working in unfamiliar surroundings or with a new team might well feel anxious too. Recognise that these feelings are normal; then deal with them so they don't have an adverse effect on your communication with patients and colleagues.

Substance abuse

The use of illegal stimulants will put your registration and your career, as well as your patients, at risk, but legal substances can also impair your performance at work. Alcohol is the main legal culprit, but prescription drugs and even some over-the-counter remedies can adversely affect performance.

- If you have a substance-abuse problem, inform your employer and seek professional help to turn your situation around.

- Be aware of the effects of legal alcohol consumption. Do not over-indulge close to a shift, and do not drink alcohol at all if you are on duty or on call.

■ Consider any side effects of prescribed medication that you are taking, and its effect on your ability to communicate and other vital aspects of your work.

Talking too much

Some people talk too much. Do you? Effective communication requires not only talking, but listening too. (Find out more about listening skills in Chapter 4.) If you talk at clients, or talk too much, it is likely that you will not be listening sufficiently or observing their facial expressions and other body language, from which you can learn so much about how they are really feeling. The more you talk, the less time there is for the other person to share in, contribute to and develop the conversation. This may leave them feeling that they do not have a stake in the exchange and they may switch off. At that point, you are no longer communicating, because they are no longer listening.

Communication should involve both parties, although not necessarily in equal measure. There are circumstances where it can be appropriate for one side to talk more than the other. When you have a lot of information to impart, you may end up doing most of the talking. In other situations, such as during counselling, or when seeking information, you may expect the client to speak most. There is no prescribed talking-to-listening ratio. Just remain sensitive to the other party and alert to the appropriate balance of talking and listening for the situation.

Why might practitioners talk too much? There are some people who love talking. If you're one of them, try to monitor yourself to ensure that you do not talk too much at work. There are occasions when any of us might find ourselves talking excessively, such as when we are nervous or embarrassed. Other situations where we may talk too much include when faced with people who we perceive to be higher in status (although this can also have the opposite effect and render us mute); when we lack confidence in our clinical skill or knowledge and try to talk our way through; when others appear to be demanding or threatening; or when there is a difficult subject to broach. Recognise the situations where you talk too much.

Reflection

Consider situations at work in which you are prone to talking too much. What are those settings and what can you do to restore a better balance between talking and listening?

If talking too much is inappropriate, talking over people is completely unacceptable. It is disrespectful, rude, aggressive and unprofessional. If an encounter is difficult or challenging, find other ways of dealing with it. Might better preparation help avert difficulties before they arise? Perhaps by anticipating the likely reaction to what you are going to say, you can manage it better. Think about how you can end difficult conversations before they start, so that you never have to talk over someone. For more techniques, read Chapters 6 and 7.

Inappropriate chat can also be a problem. Maintain a professional boundary between you and the patient, in which sharing personal talk is not appropriate. The patient might be interested in what you did at the pub last night, or what the hairdresser in the salon told you, but keep those anecdotes for outside work – or for the staff canteen. Even references to family, such as 'My auntie had the same healthcare problem as you,' may serve to trivialise the patient's condition, as their individual circumstances are most likely not the same as your friend/relative – and in any case, your auntie is irrelevant to the patient. You are there to care for the patient, not to compare them with your family members.

True story

When I was an inpatient, I overheard two nurses laughing and chatting loudly about their weekend – just the usual family and social events that most of us undertake when not working. I regarded the interaction, in working hours and within clear earshot of patients, as unprofessional, and as a result, the nurses' professional standing was diminished in my eyes.

External stresses and pressures

Events outside of work may preoccupy a practitioner's thoughts and can get in the way of effective communication. Whatever domestic or external pressures you face, the sign of a professional is the ability to leave them at the door when they arrive at work. When on duty, the service user's concerns come first. Immersing oneself in work can provide respite from any turmoil that may be experienced in one's personal life, but if external worries are interfering with your ability to communicate with, care for and support clients, then you are no longer fit for duty and must act to remedy the situation. Speak to your line manager, mentor, supervisor, occupational health counsellor or GP. Explain what is worrying you and seek help before it causes damage – to you or to others.

Boredom

Have you ever experienced that infuriating situation at a social event where the person with whom you are talking keeps looking at his or her watch, or glancing over your shoulder to see who else is in the room? It's a horrible feeling knowing that your companion is bored in your company and seeking a more stimulating chat with someone else. If you are bored at work, and convey this (intentionally, or more likely, unintentionally), it will damage the therapeutic relationship you have with your client. They will not want to share their worries, ask their questions or seek to have their anxieties addressed. It may cause them harm and delay their recovery or damage their future relationships with other practitioners in health and social care.

We may all get bored for short periods, but it is vital that this is not communicated and that we remain alert and interested in our patient. If you are experiencing long periods of disaffection or boredom at work, seek solutions such as peer counselling, or mentoring, because you will ultimately be putting your patients at risk. If that fails, you may need to ask yourself honestly whether you are in the right profession.

Chapter 3: Non-verbal communication and unintentional communication

This chapter explains how to use positive body language and other forms of non-verbal communication to enhance the patient experience and how to avoid negative body language. It also examines how unintentional communication can manifest itself and presents a practical template to enable a systematic assessment of non-verbal factors that can have an adverse impact on patients.

It is impossible not to communicate in an interaction. Even when silent, we still transmit messages – whether deliberately or accidentally. For example, think about the potentially unsettling effect of a long pause during a phone conversation. Even how you sit in a chair during a consultation can convey so much, before you've even uttered a word. The practitioner who stands when a client enters and steps forward with a welcoming smile and a gesture to take a seat is in stark contrast to the colleague who slouches back in their chair clicking a biro or chewing on a pencil, barely acknowledging that a patient has arrived. This kind of communication – the non-verbal kind – can often be more powerful than any words that are exchanged.

The Nursing and Midwifery Council's Code[34] identifies non-verbal communication as a tool to be used in an appropriate and positive manner, stating that

---

34 NMC Code (2015) *Professional Standards of Practice and Behaviour for Nurses and Midwives.* Available at: https://www.nmc.org.uk/globalassets/sitedocuments/nmc-publications/nmc-code.pdf (accessed February 2017).

practitioners should 'use a range of verbal and non-verbal communication methods, and consider cultural sensitivities, to better understand and respond to people's personal and health needs'.

The power of non-verbal communication – and the reason that healthcare practitioners need to be aware of it – is that it can add to our message; emphasise and reinforce it; substitute for verbal communication; or undermine the spoken word. When the message revealed by someone's non-verbal communication contradicts what they're saying, their message may not be believed. Positive words can be undone by negative body language. The practitioner/patient relationship can be damaged, and health may suffer. Equally, a friendly smile or appropriate eye contact can do a great deal to build rapport and trust.

So, what do we mean by the terms 'verbal communication', 'non-verbal communication' and 'unintentional communication'?

- Verbal communication is communication that uses words – written or spoken. Spoken words can be said face-to-face, over the phone or using telemedicine technology. The act of speaking or writing is deliberate, but we may still communicate unintentional messages using words. Our tone of voice can suggest an underlying irritability, thus involuntarily revealing the true feelings we have tried to mask with our friendly enquiry as to someone's well-being.

- Non-verbal communication does not use words; it involves the transmission of messages (consciously or unconsciously) using body language (bodily gestures and facial expressions).

- Unintentional communication is the transmission of an unintended message, often without the knowledge of the transmitter, or a message that is different to the intended one. This can occur using words or non-verbals. Inanimate objects can also communicate messages about us: a messy doctor's surgery or dishevelled uniform can send negative messages.

Typical example: Unintentional non-verbal communication

Vijay visits his GP for a routine check-up for high blood pressure. He's worried about anal bleeding and decides to mention it to the doctor. He walks into the consulting room, where the doctor is busy at her computer. She doesn't look up as Vijay enters. After a few seconds, having finished her typing, in a friendly tone she invites Vijay to take a seat. She tidies away a pile of paperwork as he settles himself. Vijay concludes that the doctor is too busy and that he won't 'waste' her time with his 'silly' fears. The consultation proceeds and he thanks the doctor. She feels that the consultation went well.

The doctor is unaware that by typing as Vijay entered, and clearing away paperwork, she gave the impression that she was very busy – too busy to deal with anything over and above the primary purpose of the consultation. Vijay felt unable to raise his worries about rectal bleeding with her. He may not speak to her about this concern until it is too late and his condition is untreatable. A simple miscommunication can sometimes have devastating consequences.

Verbal communication

Verbal communication can be oral (spoken) or written (this chapter focuses on spoken words; the written word will be examined in Chapter 8). Verbal communication concerns not just our choice of words – the vocabulary we select when we speak or write – but also how something is said. Does the tone or volume match the message? Have we used friendly words but an irritable pitch? Have we emphasised one word or phrase above others, to reinforce it?

Tone, pitch, volume, pauses, fluency and speed of speech – collectively known as 'paralinguistics' – are all factors that can lend additional meaning to our choice of words. Someone who says that they are happy to discuss any concerns, then speeds on to the next subject without pausing, is communicating that they don't really have the time or the inclination. The failure to pause creates an unspoken message that contradicts the message conveyed in the chosen words. The person who replies 'yes' after a long pause indicates that they may not be fully in agreement. Someone who loudly announces that you can share a confidence with them might well give the impression that they cannot be trusted to keep it quiet. A normally fluent person who pauses and 'ums' and 'ahs' may convey that s/he is distracted or nervous about something. Someone who is short and curt in responses, often using just a single word by way of reply ('perhaps,' 'possibly', 'no'), could be showing that they are not fully engaged in a conversation, or that they are angry, cynical or fed up.

Typically, face-to-face communication involves the interaction between spoken words and body language – and the 'decoding' of these by the recipient – resulting in the transmission of intended and unintended messages. In any interaction, you will 'read' clients and interpret what is said and how it is said, in conjunction with body language and other non-verbal signs; patients in turn will read you. This may happen consciously or unconsciously.

Reflection

Say the word 'quickly' aloud in front of a mirror, in a neutral way. Now say it in angry or irritated fashion. Now adopt a friendly and encouraging manner when you say it. Now sound nervous. Did your face change at all? How did your voice change? Be aware of what you convey when you speak – over and above the words. Do you sound like you are in a hurry? Might this deter patients from sharing their concerns? Do you have a sharp tone that comes across as fierce, making you unapproachable? Are you too softly spoken, so that your intelligent and well-considered observations lack gravitas with colleagues? Reflect on the way you speak, and ask friends, family and colleagues for honest feedback. Do you need to make any adjustments? Think about someone whose communication style you admire. Reflect on the techniques they employ.

Non-verbal communication

Non-verbal communication is primarily about body language, but other factors can also communicate a message, such as the layout or decoration of a room or the dress or appearance of the speaker. A warm and restful waiting area can communicate a welcoming message; conversely an untidy, harshly-lit reception room can do the opposite. These often unintentional messages will be explored in greater detail in the section below on unintentional communication.

Body language is a complex interplay between various factors, such as:

- **Position:** how we position our bodies (folding our arms or inclining our head, for example); and proxemics or 'personal space' (where and how close/apart we position ourselves to others).

- **Facial expressions:** smiles, frowns and raised eyebrows, for example.

- **Eye contact:** whether we look at others, and how we do it (staring, looking away, sideways, or over someone's shoulder).

- **Touch:** how and where we touch ourselves, others, and objects (such as our glasses, clothing or pens).

- **Physical reactions:** such as perspiring, blushing or breathing rapidly.

Various claims are made about the percentage that can be attributed to the impact of non-verbal communication versus words. The figure quoted varies wildly, and is generally unhelpful. Each encounter is unique, and the effect of any non-verbal communication will be individual to each situation. It will be affected by factors such as:

- How someone is generally regarded: people might be more tolerant of negative body language from someone who is widely regarded as brusque, for example, than from a person who is usually very kind and helpful (that's not to say that it is acceptable to be terse or abrupt all the time).

- The recipient's sensitivities: each individual will react differently. Some people are more sensitive than others. Sensitivities are not static, and may change according to the situation.

- The situation: there might be greater sensitivity to non-verbal communication in emotionally charged situations, such as those that many practitioners have to deal with.

Non-verbal communication will have a significant effect in conversations with patients and colleagues, and as such, it needs to be considered.

Research[35] has shown a relationship between non-verbal behaviour and patient perceptions of a clinician's empathy. Eye contact and social touch (such as a handshake or a pat on the back) significantly enhanced the interaction for the patient, who felt that the clinician was more empathetic. (Other studies have also found eye contact between the clinician and the patient significantly boosted patient ratings of rapport and satisfaction.) The researchers concluded that clinical environments designed for patient and clinician interaction should be designed to facilitate positive non-verbal interactions such as eye contact and social touch. (Practitioners report that appropriate touch can positively enhance an encounter, but caution should always be exercised when using it. Touch could be misinterpreted as being too intimate, even sexual, or just plain condescending. It can also create difficulties if socially or culturally inappropriate. Even ritualistic touch, such as shaking hands as a form of greeting, can be culturally unacceptable in certain circumstances. Always consider asking permission before touching, including for task-related touching such as taking blood pressure or pulse.)

Body language is a two-way process. We transmit messages to others; and we receive and interpret meaning from other people's body language. Understanding body language will help you to use it in a more self-aware way to:

- aid communication

- avoid unconscious messages which could be harmful to relationships

- decode and react appropriately to other people's visual cues.

---

35 Montague E, Chen P, Xu J, Chewning B & Barrett B (2013) Nonverbal interpersonal interactions in clinical encounters and patient perceptions of empathy. *Journal of Participatory Medicine* **5** e33.

Body language is often regarded as a set of subconscious actions that give away what we really think or feel, but it can also be a positive tool that can be used deliberately to reinforce the spoken word and to build rapport. In a therapeutic relationship, body language can be used to help you understand how a client is really feeling. Someone who says that they are fine might be betrayed by body language indicating that the opposite is true. Being alert to body language can enable you to probe a little deeper, rather than simply accepting a verbal response at face value. If you explain a procedure and the patient looks worried (frowning, or avoiding eye contact, for example) but says nothing, you might wish to reassure by stating that it is natural to be worried and to invite questions about any fears they may have. Or indeed simply the way they are holding themselves or their stance might be indicative of pain or discomfort they are not revealing. 'Reading' a client's body language will help you to give them better support. It can be as important as observing their clinical symptoms.

Be careful not to misinterpret body language and reach the wrong conclusions. Triangulate information from different sources to form a holistic picture. Listen to what patients say, and consider what you know about them from personal knowledge or their health records, rather than relying on body language as your sole source. Also consider body language in the round, looking at clusters or combinations of behaviours rather than focusing on a single indicator. For example, a sweating patient may be nervous – or just hot, suffering from diabetes, hypertension or the menopause. You might be on safer ground in concluding that it's nerves rather than heat if the sweating is combined with an avoidance of eye contact and the wringing of hands. (Observing a patient's body language can also enable you to pick up symptoms that can form part of the clinical picture. Sweating may indicate an infection, for example.)

Also be alert to cultural and other differences. How close to each other we stand or sit varies across cultures. 'Proxemics' is the codification of personal space into distinctly different 'distance zones' (intimate, personal, social and public), depending on the nature of the relationship. We generally allow those with whom we have intimate or personal relationships – such as sexual partners, or close friends – to stand or sit closer to us than we would allow the general public (although in certain situations, such as on a crowded underground train, we may tolerate strangers being closer to us than we would otherwise accept). Discomfort can occur when someone's personal space is 'invaded', and conversely also when we feel that the distance is inappropriately large. You may be the creator of the discomfort, or the recipient. In clinical situations, you may need to enter someone's personal or even intimate zone, and this can create discomfort or embarrassment in itself, regardless of any cultural differences. Try to be sensitive to this. It can sometimes help simply to acknowledge how someone might be feeling, and how normal that feeling is: 'No one likes this, but don't worry. It won't take long.'

Body language can vary across different age groups. There may be gender differences too, such as the use of touch as a form of communication. However, remember that there are some basic human emotions – such as fear, anger and sadness – which tend to present themselves universally (in terms of our facial expressions), regardless of factors such as culture, age or social class.

Body language dos and don'ts

- Don't use negative body language such as folding your arms or crossing your legs; poor posture when standing or sitting (slumped shoulders suggest a lack of confidence and self-worth, which may undermine your professional credibility); wringing your hands; holding a palm up towards a patient, indicating 'stop'; playing with a pen or other item, indicating that you are distracted or nervous.

- Do look for opportunities to use positive body language – such as smiling when greeting someone, leaning forward rather than slumping back, inclining your head when listening, and making appropriate eye contact.

- Don't stifle a yawn, or keep looking towards the door/at your phone/at the clock – it suggests that you wish to bring a consultation to an end. If you do need to leave, or to draw a session to a close, use words: 'I'm sorry, but we have run out of time for this week …' (Consider setting expectations at the outset: 'We need to finish by 2pm today.')

- Do bring yourself to the same physical level as a patient, both to ease communication and to ensure that you do not transmit an unintentional message about status.

- Don't automatically assume that someone who is not making eye contact with you is 'shifty' or being untruthful. In some cultures, direct eye contact is considered rude and not making eye contact may be a sign of respect. Some people with conditions such as Asperger syndrome may find eye contact uncomfortable or even invasive and will keep their eyes down, or focus on something other than the speaker.

- Do look out for 'micro gestures', such as the slightest raising of an eyebrow. Even when someone is trying hard to control their body language, these very small signs can indicate how they are really feeling.

- Don't confuse meaning. Someone who is biting their lip may be anxious, or just concentrating. Ask open questions to confirm: 'How are you feeling?'

- Do remember that body language is but one indicator, and other factors should also be considered. Look out for disparities between what is said and what you observe. Someone who shrugs their shoulders dismissively and pronounces: 'Oh, it doesn't matter' might be betrayed by body language that suggests that actually it does matter a great deal.

Unintentional communication

From time to time, we all – practitioners and patients – transmit a message that is at odds with the one we believe we're communicating. It can be the root cause of many misunderstandings in life – including in healthcare settings. By learning to avoid our own unintentional communication, and by recognising and learning to read patients' unintentional messages, we can build a better rapport and create a stronger therapeutic relationship.

Social leakage

When we speak, generally we pay attention only to our chosen words. When we listen to others speak, we experience the interaction in the round, observing body language, and noticing volume, pace and pitch of the spoken word too. Humans are very good at picking up any dissonance between these. Someone who is tapping their foot or drumming their fingers may give the impression that they are irritated or impatient, regardless of any spoken words of reassurance to the contrary. This is known as 'social leakage' – our unconscious actions betraying our conscious words. Even the most fleeting, most subtle glance at the clock will be detected, or the slightest quaver in one's voice. Such visual and audible messages, of which the healthcare professional may be oblivious, could deter a patient from continuing to elaborate on their concerns. That is why we need to learn to recognise ways in which we may deliver negative messages, so that we can avoid them.

Unintentional messages may be carried by:

■ body language (posture, eye contact, facial expressions, gestures, and so on)

■ how we speak (tone, pace, volume, pitch – and even accent)

■ our appearance (clothing, hair)

■ environmental factors (surroundings such as the consulting room or office).

Reflection

Think of a situation with a friend or family member where they said one thing, but you believed them to mean another. Analyse the interaction. Identify specifically what made you feel that they meant something different to what they said. Was it tone of voice? Body language? Consciously observe other people's body language – patients' and colleagues' – and learn to be aware of your own too, particularly in situations that you find difficult. Self-awareness may help you to alter or control your body language if/where necessary.

The Figure 1.2 (in Chapter 1) shows factors that could interfere with a practitioner's message, resulting in it reaching patients in an altered form. Figure 3.1 illustrates how practitioners can inadvertently communicate a very different message to the one they think they are transmitting.

Figure 3.1: Communicating unintentional messages.

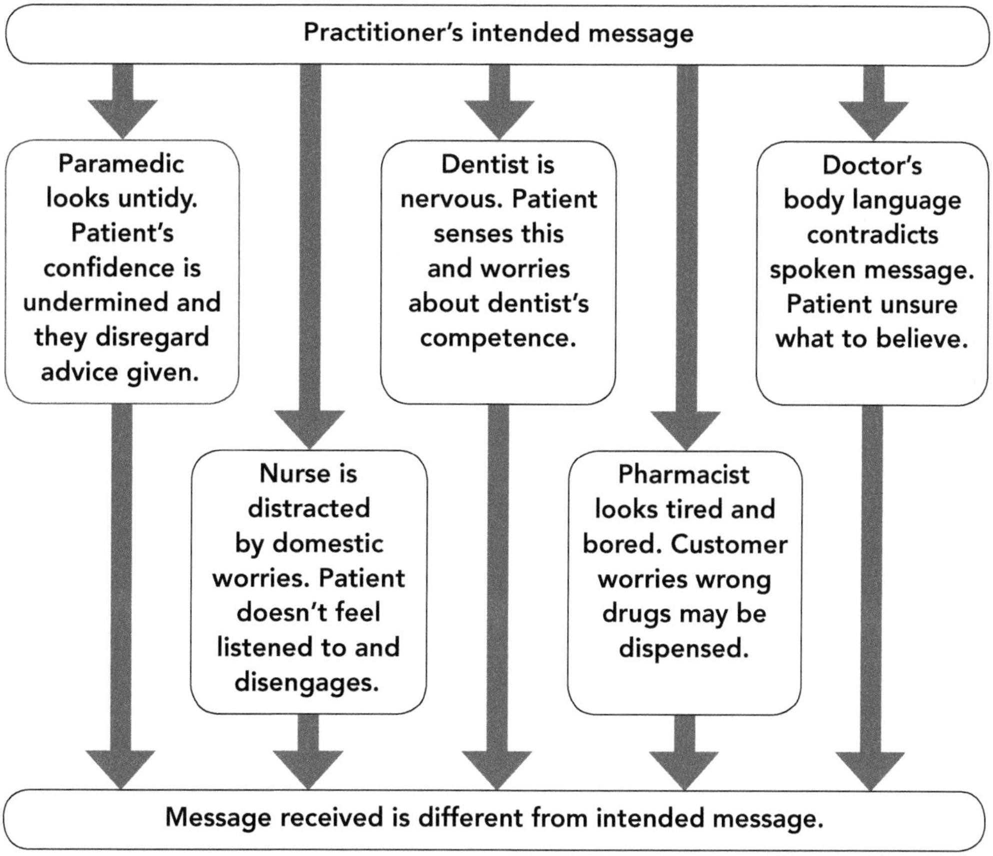

There was once a time when healthcare professionals were assigned almost automatic trust. Those days of deference are largely gone, and many patients are less likely to unquestioningly accept something merely because a doctor or a nurse says that it is the case. Clients will form an assessment about professional credibility based on various factors. If credibility is undermined for some reason, the impact of your message will be diluted.

Appearance

Whether or not we should judge a book by its cover, or a person by their appearance, regrettably it does happen. Whether we're fat or thin, black or white, attractive or plain, flamboyant or dowdy, the way we look can be a powerful communicator of intentional and unintentional messages. There are aspects of our appearance that we have control over, such as our hairstyle or body piercings, and others – such as skin colour – that we do not. People's prejudices can affect how we are regarded. Assumptions will be made about our status and intelligence on the basis of our ethnicity, gender or age, for example. We must be careful not to make any such prejudgements about our patients.

Uniformed practitioners such as paramedics or white-coated doctors can convey a certain power and authority that they may not communicate when in normal dress. This may evoke deference and compliance in some patients, particularly from certain groups. Body piercings and tattoos may convey credibility in some settings and for some groups of service users, and negative messages for others. The same goes for business attire. It can suggest authority or professionalism to some; stuffiness to others. Dress appropriately for the occasion.

Be conscious of your physical appearance and how others may react to you as a result. What does your style of dress say about you? Do you have any choice over what to wear, or must you adhere to the specified uniform or your organisation's dress code? In my local children's hospice, clinical staff don't wear uniforms because that would be at odds with the homely atmosphere they wish to create so that families feel relaxed. Whether you wear a uniform or not, appropriate dress for your professional role will help you establish credibility with clients.

Environmental factors

The waiting room with out-of-date, dog-eared magazines; the harshly illuminated, pictureless consulting room; the dimly lit, grey-painted hospital corridor; the gloomy dental surgery with pop music blaring from the radio; the smelly nursing home with mismatched chairs; or the shabby office crammed with dusty medical books – they all convey strong unintentional messages. Professor Dianne Berry[36] stressed that it is 'important to ensure that a room's layout and so on will facilitate rather than impede effective communication'.

The care provided in an institution may be first class, but if it is let down by poor surroundings, it may be perceived as less than good. Conversely, restful,

36 Berry D (2007) *Health Communication: Theory and Practice*. Maidenhead: Open University Press.

thoughtfully designed or attractively laid-out surroundings can have a positive impact on patients' well-being. Small touches – a bunch of flowers, a pretty picture, a pleasant fragrance – can have a big impact, because they communicate that you care. Think about what patients might need, and try to ensure that they are provided. Clients may expect a place to hang their clothes and handbag, and a mirror to check their appearance before emerging from a cubicle after dressing. If fashion retailers' changing rooms provide these basic facilities, surely the NHS can too! They are really important considerations, which are often absent even in places where they should be obvious, such as in breast-surgery clinics.

Patient-centric organisations

Organisations striving for excellent client service value positive communication and recognise the potentially negative effect of unintentional communication. They can see the aggregate impact on patients of small things that go wrong. A little thing here and an even tinier thing there, taken individually, are just annoying; cumulatively they can add up to a great deal of upset. Whether it's a patient left waiting and no one telling them what's happening, or a clinician getting a client's name wrong, these communication failures are exacerbated when service users are feeling anxious or stressed – which is often the case in healthcare. If you are a leader in your organisation, take notice of the opportunities for unintentional communication to occur and do something about it.

True story

My mother was admitted to a nursing home. Desperately worried, we drove 250 miles through terrible weather to see her. She was being prepared for bed when we arrived, so we were shown into a small room to wait. It had no windows, and the fluorescent tube threw out a cold, harsh light. The room doubled-up as a store cupboard, its floor-to-ceiling shelving storing toilet rolls and incontinence pads. There were two mismatched chairs and three of us needing seats. We weren't even offered a cup of tea after our long journey. This experience communicated a very powerful message to me, namely that my mother was not in a caring place and that I needed to find an alternative nursing home urgently. It transpired that the home was acceptable, and she remained a resident there, but that experience communicated quite a different message that could have resulted in my moving her to another home.

Consider carrying out a workplace audit to assess unintentional communication. It's not difficult. Use the practical template below (Template 3.1), which can be adapted to evaluate any type of workplace, be it a clinic, ward or other environment. The audit template will help you to see your workplace as patients and other important stakeholders see it. It will enable you to identify unintentional communication and, crucially, it will help you to adopt a systematic approach to reducing it. Of course, it is impossible to eradicate all unintentional communication, but the tool will go a long way to creating a more positive atmosphere, with less negative unintentional communication.

Template 3.1: Unintentional communications audit template

Item	What it communicates about us	What we'd like to communicate	Required action	Owner	Budget	Deadline

Conducting an unintentional communications audit is simple. Begin by thinking about how unintentional messages may be carried, and draw up a list. Use this list to populate the first column in the template (a completed sample template can be seen on the next page – Template 3.2). What you include will vary from organisation to organisation, but might include:

- *Website / printed information:* What do your publications (patient information leaflets, annual report etc.) and website say about you – not just the words, but the images, ease of use, and so on? What would you think about your workplace if you saw these things and had no other knowledge on which to base your view? Look at the content, but also at the kind of language used and what message that conveys. Anything over-wordy, pompous or full of jargon will convey negative messages, whereas patients will welcome clear, concise, plain English communications. What messages are conveyed by your choice of photographs or illustrations? Is a good cross section of the community represented? Is there an overemphasis on pictures of staff? Review your website and printed materials.

- *Notices and signs:* Sometimes notices and signs can let down an otherwise caring organisation. Officious, unfriendly signs communicate negative messages. Take a look at notices and check that they do not hector, lecture or order visitors: 'Mobile phones not allowed,' 'No smoking on hospital premises,' 'We will not tolerate assaults on staff,' and so on. These may be legitimate messages, but express them in a friendly, helpful or explanatory style. Remove unnecessary notices and reword necessary ones where appropriate ('Please wash your hands' rather than 'Now wash your hands').

- *Correspondence:* The written word is as important as the spoken word. Check your organisation's standardised letters to see if they communicate any unintentional messages. Are letters and emails officious and impersonal in style, or lacking the human touch? Might they make the reader feel that you don't care, or don't see them as an individual? Can they be improved? (See Chapter 8 for more information.)

- *Client welcome:* Do clients receive a warm welcome from a friendly, helpful receptionist or must they settle for a grunt and a nod? Front-line staff such as receptionists and telephonists are fundamental to a positive patient experience. Observe interactions, get feedback from visitors, and decide whether training is required.

- *Phone manner:* Consider asking a 'mystery shopper', such as a friend or relative, to call your organisation to assess what message is communicated by the way calls are handled. Listen in on speaker-phone to assess whether the switchboard/receptionist is helpful, knowledgeable and professional. Is the caller put through to the right extension first time, or their query answered correctly? Reflect on how a similar experience would leave a patient feeling. What does it communicate about your workplace?

■ *Premises:* What do your premises look like from outside? What message will clients receive before they get through the door? Once inside, is the reception area comfortable and welcoming? Piles of dog-eared copies of the People's Friend from 2009, and posters for events that have long since taken place, communicate an out-of-touch organisation. A pleasant environment can put patients at ease. Decent waiting, office and consulting space can be achieved on limited means with a bit of imagination – even on an NHS budget. Good premises communicate a positive message to those using your service.

Look at all aspects of your clinic/surgery/workplace that have a potential for communicating negative messages to users. Be wary of relying solely on your own perceptions. Get a true picture by asking patients for their views. Consider sending out an anonymous questionnaire to elicit honest feedback. Talk to service users and find out what they think about you – either through focus groups or as part of a hospital walkabout. Many NHS organisations used walkabouts to chat to service users and to identify improvements based on user feedback. Use suggestions/comment boxes to gather input, or write asking clients what they think. Complaints are another source of useful information. By looking critically at your workplace through others' eyes, you can introduce improvements and become a better organisation when it comes to communicating and listening.

Template 3.2: Sample completed unintentional communications audit template

Item	What it communicates about us	What we'd like to communicate	Required action	Owner	Budget	Deadline
Patient leaflet on our service.	Makes us appear authoritarian and unhelpful – too much about rules and regulations rather than what we can do for the patient. Language too clinical/technical.	Friendly, responsive service structured around patient needs.	Rewrite in a more friendly style using plain English. Ensure we convey that we are a patient-centric organisation.	Jackie Smith.	N/A as leaflet due for a refresh and already budgeted for.	July 1st.

Reception.	Dreary, cold and unwelcoming – gives the impression that we don't care about patients' comfort.	Calm, comfortable and relaxing, without looking expensive. We want clients to feel welcome and relaxed.	Repaint in sunny lemon. Hang framed drawings by local school children. Play calming classical music. Buy pot plants.	Maintenance manager to arrange painting. Stewart to organise other actions.	£800.	ASAP but no later than July 16th.
Website.	Suggests that we are not a diverse organisation – all images are of white, able-bodied staff/patients.	That we have a diverse workforce and community and respect difference.	Replace images with photos that better reflect diversity of our community.	Amina and website designer.	N/A as can be done in-house.	June 30th.
Telephones.	Pick-up is too slow; style is brusque as staff are busy; no recorded message for after-hours calls. Gives impression that we don't care about clients' calls.	Helpful, friendly, caring – we welcome calls from clients and want to handle them professionally and com-passionately.	Davie to work on switchboard 9am–10am (peak times) to improve call pick-up by boosting staffing levels. Training for staff on switchboard. Record friendly message asking callers to call back between 9am and 5pm when clinic is open. Set up voicemail so messages can be left out of hours.	Sue to revise staffing rotas to allow Davie to be on switchboard. Arif to organise training and voicemail message.	Speak to HR dept. to confirm costs of training (internal?) and overtime costs to backfill rotas during training.	August 20th.

Dos and don'ts for effective face-to-face communication

- Do pay special attention to your own verbal and non-verbal communication on first meeting a client, as first impressions can be hard to shake off.

- Don't allow a messy desk or untidy personal dress to inadvertently communicate a poor impression. Pay attention to how you and your workplace look.

- Do learn to read patients' body language, as it can help you identify how they are really feeling.

- Don't overlook the importance of a conducive environment for service user interactions. Do what you can to create an appropriate atmosphere.

Chapter 4: Effective listening, observing and questioning

Listening and observing are as important as speaking. Effective communication cannot take place without them. This chapter offers practical tips on active listening and demonstrates the importance of observing patients' reactions. Key techniques covered include asking questions to seek information – and checking and clarifying answers.

Talking takes effort, and so does listening. It's not a passive act, in which our ears are always open and 'switched on', with words just drifting from the speaker's mouth into the listener's ear. Listening requires active brainwork and genuine engagement. Words need to be heard, considered and digested. Reactions must be observed – meaning that active listening requires ears and eyes. Most of us are not as good at it as we think we are.

Research suggests that much of the time we fail to hear a percentage of what is said, and just a short time after a conversation, can recall as little as a quarter to a half of what we were told. One healthcare study found that just five minutes after a consultation, patients had forgotten half of what they had been told. Patients' poor recall means that they are less likely to comply with medical advice, which may result in adverse outcomes for them. (See the end of this chapter for tips on how to help improve patients' recall.) For practitioners, inattention also leads to poor recall, and this too can result in poorer outcomes for patients.

Why is listening essential? For the healthcare practitioner, listening is important because it is a principal way of gathering information about a client's condition or symptoms (whether direct from the patient or via a colleague or patient's relative) so that the correct care and treatment can be provided. The practitioner can ask questions to get the patient's history, but we only get the information we need if we listen to and probe the answers given.

For the patient, being listened to is important if trust and rapport are to be established with the healthcare practitioner. Patients need to know that they are being heard. Otherwise, what is the point in speaking? Think about how you feel when you're just not being listened to. It can be infuriating, demoralising, diminishing … However it makes you feel, the emotion is likely to be a negative one. Not being heard can be damaging; conversely, being heard can have a positive impact. Even outside a formal counselling scenario, patients can derive great therapeutic value from being listened to and understood.

Reflection

Think about a time when you told someone something important to you, but you felt that you were just not listened to. What made you believe that you weren't being heard? How did it make you feel? How did you react? How do you want patients to feel when they speak with you? What do you need to do differently to ensure that they feel the way you would like them to feel?

'Mindfulness' has proved to be a useful tool for helping people to be conscious of the present moment – the right here, right now. Too often, external distractions (noise, other people) and internal diversions (thoughts or worries) take us away from the present moment. Learning to shut these out will enable you to focus on patients and listen actively to them. Mindful listening:

- improves retention (so you will be able to remember more of what is said)

- increases attention span (so you stay alert for longer)

- improves understanding (which enhances rapport)

- reduces error (which improves accuracy and boosts patient safety).

Mindful, active listening involves consciously hearing what someone is saying to you, paying special attention throughout the encounter, and observing body language in order fully to understand what the service user is communicating. To consciously hear, silence your own inner thoughts. If you are preoccupied thinking about the next task (or what you're going to cook for dinner), it will interfere with your ability to focus wholly on your patient's message.

Barriers to listening

Students and newly qualified practitioners can find that they're so absorbed in concentrating on what they are doing, and trying to get it right, that they end up only half-listening.

Experienced healthcare practitioners can sometimes find themselves in a kind of 'autopilot' mode, where a certain procedure has been done so many times before that they just perform it without really thinking about it or observing reactions – taking a blood sample, for example, or some other routine task. You might make 'small talk' while undertaking such a procedure, almost absent-mindedly saying the same thing to every patient – such as commenting on the weather – while your thoughts are on other matters, work or domestic. Small talk can be important in building trust and putting patients at ease, but the practitioner needs to remain alert, really listen to the patient's responses and observe their reactions.

It is easy to forget that something you've done a hundred or even a thousand times could well be the first time for your patient. They may have questions to ask, feel anxious, or need reassurance. Unless you are mindfully there with them, listening and observing, a patient's feelings and concerns could simply pass you by. This will lead to a poorer patient experience and could result in poorer treatment if important cues are overlooked.

The expression 'to give one's undivided attention' is a useful one to reflect upon, because all too often we offer our divided attention. Consider what you can do to minimise or eradicate distractions that result in only a proportion of your attention being dedicated to your patient. You will inevitably be distracted if the computer in the consulting room pings each time an email arrives (or your mobile phone vibrates in your pocket). If you're wondering who's making contact, the connection between you and your patient will suffer.

Distractions come in many shapes and forms. Learn to recognise what interferes with your attention. It might be something about the patient, such as the way they dress, their accent or their mannerisms. Do not allow such things to affect your listening. Learn to block them out and to listen without judging or mentally criticising.

If you are due to have an important conversation with a service user, try to take a moment immediately beforehand to clear your head of potential distractions. Try to leave domestic worries at home when you are at work, so that they cannot preoccupy you and divert attention from the people you are being paid to care for.

Take several deep breaths, mentally switch off from other cares and concerns, and make a commitment to offer your full attention.

Another barrier to effective listening is our ability to block messages we don't like or feel uncomfortable about, or things we would rather not hear because they are difficult to deal with. Sometimes we subconsciously filter them out so that we don't have to face them, talk about them, or address them. As a professional, you cannot simply mentally ignore what a patient says. Become conscious of situations where you are prone to block messages and choose to actively listen instead. And always be mindful of the possibility that your patient is blocking out the difficult message which you may be trying to deliver.

Checking and clarifying

One of the principal ways of gathering information is by asking questions – and listening to the answers. It sounds so easy, but what someone says and what we hear may not be the same thing. We interpret what has been heard through our own lens of knowledge, experience, prejudices and beliefs. These things about us affect how we react to what is being said, which in turn affects what we hear (and what we don't hear). Learn to recognise the factors that influence how you hear and interpret/reinterpret. Set prejudices aside.

Misunderstandings can arise as a result of us incorrectly interpreting what was said, or through an unclear or incomplete account being provided that leaves gaps in our understanding. That is why it is important that we check that we have correctly heard what was said. Summarise, recap, paraphrase or ask questions to check or clarify. This gives the patient an opportunity to correct any misunderstanding: 'You have told me that you have had swollen, tender knees for two months now – the left knee being more painful than the right. You are finding it difficult to manage stairs too. Is that right? Have I missed anything?'

Useful phrases for checking and clarifying include:

■ 'Can I just check that I've understood this correctly? You have said that ...'

■ 'Let me check that I'm clear about your symptoms. You tell me that ...'

■ 'I want to be sure I understand what you mean ...'

■ 'What you seem to be saying is ...'

■ 'Could you tell me more about ...'

■ 'Have I got that summary right, or is there anything I've missed?'

Be prepared for patients to correct your summary. Listen to any corrections respectfully and without being defensive. Your aim is to improve your understanding. Continue in this vein until you are sure that your understanding is accurate.

Dos and don'ts of active listening

- Do look at the patient, focus on what they are saying, and concentrate on their message.
- Don't allow what's happening around you to distract you. Screen out other activity and background noise.
- Do pay attention and demonstrate that you are listening by nodding, and so on.
- Don't get bored, drift off or daydream. If you find that happening, consciously refocus.
- Do encourage the speaker to continue, by giving an occasional smile or other appropriate reinforcing body language.
- Don't think about how you're going to respond or rehearse what you're going to say next, as this will distract you from listening.

Everyone wants to be heard, but listening alone is not enough: show that you are listening too. Simply incline your head, nod or make occasional affirmative sounds, like 'mm' or 'uh huh'. This serves to acknowledge that you are listening attentively. Vary your response throughout the conversation, as a robotic stream of 'uh huhs' may have the counter effect. Be warm and natural, as a mechanistic response sounds insincere.

Reflection

Have a conversation with a friend or colleague in which your friend sits with his/her back to you so there is no eye contact. Does this have a positive, negative or neutral effect on the interaction? Ask your friend for feedback too. Discuss how you each felt, and consider the reasons for this. What learning can you apply from this exercise?

Practitioners sometimes worry that if they say 'yes', nod, or otherwise encourage patients to speak using active listening techniques, this may make clients believe you agree with what they're saying. This can be problematic in a situation where you are being told something with which you profoundly disagree, but you're required to encourage the patient to talk in order to elicit key information. Try not to be judgemental, and remember that listening and encouraging are not the same as agreeing.

Listening can be a frustrating business when the speaker is not a good communicator. Some clients will be inarticulate, slow or hesitant in their answers; unclear, confused, contradictory or incomplete in their accounts – whether as a result of their condition, because of nervousness, or because that is their natural disposition. In such situations it can be tempting to butt in and finish a sentence or make their point for them. The lure of this must be resisted. You do not know what they are planning to say, but even if you feel sure that you do, be patient and listen respectfully. Do not jump to conclusions or wade in and suggest solutions or a way forward – until you've heard their full story. Allow people the time, space and, if necessary, encouragement to speak for themselves and to finish their account. Interruptions and interventions may make them feel that you don't have the time or inclination to listen, or that you don't value what they are saying, thus inhibiting what or how much they are willing to share with you. If you are unclear about something, wait for a natural pause in the conversation before interrupting to ask for clarification or further explanation.

Reflect on your own communications style. If someone is having difficulty in expressing themselves, might they also be struggling to understand you? Do you need to slow down a little, use a different or more appropriate vocabulary, or ask for (or provide) information in smaller chunks?

Asking questions

When you trained as a healthcare practitioner, you most likely learned how to take a clinical history. When you trained will most likely determine what you were taught about how to do this. The structured and systematic approach that is imparted to students is valuable because it ensures that all bases are covered – in theory at least. However, there is a risk that in attempting to focus in on what is wrong, questions become increasingly closed or funnelled. The richness of information that comes from open-ended enquiry may be lost. Open questions allow for more of an unstructured, free-flowing dialogue than the staccato closed Q&A format, in which a question posed by the practitioner is followed by a yes/no answer from the patient. Open questions can produce improved quality and quantity of clinical data, potentially leading to differential diagnoses and better patient outcomes. A more conversational style can also build rapport and coax patients into disclosing more information, which in turn can help with diagnosis. Patients may feel better listened to, and respond positively and openly. (There is a place for short, focused questions, such as in the emergency department, where getting information quickly may literally be a matter of life or death.)

Depending on the field of healthcare that you work in, typical open questions might include:

- What is the problem?
- What/how are you feeling?
- Why do you think you feel that way?
- Tell me about any other symptoms.
- Why do you think it might have happened?
- What were you doing that may have caused it?
- What effect does it have on your day-to-day life?

If you have a hunch as to what is wrong, it can be tempting to start asking either closed or leading questions (or both) to help confirm the diagnosis:

- Are you having trouble sleeping?
- Have you been feeling nauseous?
- Would you say you feel depressed?
- You're not constipated, are you?

Leading questions may result in answers that allow the patient an early exit from an uncomfortable consultation. Patients may be happy to be led because it's easier and quicker to say yes/no than to go into detail and offer a full account. Better alternatives would be:

- Tell me how you are sleeping.
- What symptoms have you had?
- How is your mood, or how are you feeling within yourself?
- Tell me about your bowel habits.

These open questions are neutral and do not suggest a 'right' answer. They allow for a more discursive conversation. Clinical decisions will be based to a large extent on information gathered during the patient interview, so a consultation comprising a more relaxed conversational style will encourage the patient to relax, open up, and to share more information with you. In turn, this will aid more accurate diagnoses.

Questions can be used to shift the direction of the discussion. This can be positive, if the conversation is drifting off topic and needs to be refocused and brought back on track with an opportune intervention. However, be careful not to inadvertently negatively shift direction with an ill-timed or ill-considered intervention that breaks the natural flow or sends it in the wrong direction.

Improving patient recall

It is extremely common for patients to be unable to recall information they have recently been given by a health or social care practitioner. Even those who believe that they remember what they have been told quite often misremember, or simply get it wrong. For all manner of reasons – such as anxiety, pain or the effect of medicines – a patient may not be sufficiently attentive, which will affect understanding and ability to recall. Even where a patient offers their full attention, if the practitioner delivers over-complex, jargon-laden information, or offers it in huge chunks that cannot easily be digested, the message may not be understood – and even if it is, recall may be affected. It is your responsibility to help patients to receive your message and to be able to recall it accurately.

Dos and don'ts

- Do make sure patients are put at ease so they can concentrate on the message.
- Don't use technical language, as patients will not understand the message.
- Do break the message into bite-size chunks.
- Don't forget to check their understanding before moving on to the next chunk.
- Do wait until the effects of shock/drugs have worn off before providing important information, where possible.

In studies, improved client comprehension and information retention has been achieved simply by asking patients to explain to another member of the care team what they have just been told in a consultation. Any misunderstandings can be put right at this stage too.

Be mindful. Be observant. Be sensitive. Be flexible in your communication style. By improving your own listening skills, and helping patients to improve their understanding and retention, you can help improve patient outcomes and make for an all-round better experience – for you as well as for your clients.

Chapter 5: Communicating with people who have particular needs

This chapter explores practical ways of communicating effectively with a range of people who have specific or special needs, such as those with a hearing or visual impairment, dementia sufferers, people with a learning disability, or individuals whose first language is not English. The chapter also examines ways of communicating with children and young people.

In a sense we all have special needs, because each of us is unique. Everyone appreciates being treated as an individual and receiving a tailored response. That is why unthinkingly applying blanket approaches in our communications will fail. There is a common belief that older people do not like healthcare professionals using their first names – preferring instead the more formal Mr/Mrs – but an article for BMJ Open[37] suggested that ethnic and cultural factors can influence preferred modes of address too, and that research in an Irish geriatric unit found that older people there preferred first-name usage. This underlines the need to establish personal preferences. A simple check for all patients results in getting it right for each and every individual.

---

37 Parsons SR, Hughes AJ & Friedman ND (2016) 'Please don't call me Mister': patient preferences of how they are addressed and their knowledge of their treating medical team in an Australian hospital. *BMJ Open*.

True story

My name is Moiram, but I've always been known as Moi – except decades ago when I was at school. Healthcare professionals call me Moiram, the name on my notes, which makes me feel like I'm a little girl again. If only they'd ask about preferences, it would make for a much more comfortable, less grating conversation from my perspective. Another favourite is to call me Mrs Ali. As a feminist, I refused to adopt my husband's surname or the title 'Mrs', so being call Mrs Ali rather than Ms really annoys me.

In an article in the *Journal of the American Medical Association*,[38] failure to check the patient's preferred name was interpreted by a son as a lack of personal interest in his father, the patient. The author, a medic, felt uncomfortable about his father, Jack, being called by his legal name, Harold, in hospital. 'For me it has been a journey into the medical system as an inexperienced consumer rather than in my usual position as a seasoned provider … Dad never has been 'Harold', except to those who really don't know him … Dad doesn't correct his physicians or the office receptionists – he is from the old school, where it is impolite to question or correct your physician.'

The solution? Simply ask individual patients how they wish to be addressed rather than making an assumption based on the group you perceive someone to belong to.

The over-riding message is to regard each person as an individual, even though some groups of individuals may have shared communication needs. Even within a group, though, such as among people who are deaf, there will be huge variation. Younger deaf people may prefer information such as healthcare appointment reminders to be sent by text message; some older people may not even have a mobile phone, and blind people will be unable to read letters or text messages.

Some service users have multiple needs due a number of factors affecting their ability to communicate. Someone who does not speak English as a first language may also suffer from dementia and age-related hearing loss. A young person may also have a visual impairment. When it comes to sight loss, nearly two-thirds of those affected are women; and people from black and minority ethnic communities are at greater risk of some of the leading causes of sight loss. Adults with learning disabilities are ten times more likely to be blind or partially sighted than the general population. Whatever grouping someone may fall within, react to everyone as an individual and see the person first, and not any impairment or condition. You can then tailor any response to meet their specific needs.

---

38 Bruder Stapleton F (2000) My name is Jack. *Journal of the American Medical Association*, **284** (16) 2027.

The legislation

In order to be a good healthcare practitioner, and to build a strong therapeutic relationship, recognising someone's particular needs is essential. Over and above that, your organisation may also have a legal duty to cater for the information and communication needs of certain groups. The Equality Act 2010[39] (applicable in England, Scotland and Wales – Northern Ireland has similar legislation) applies to health services – including hospitals, GPs, dentists and opticians – and requires, among other things, the provision of information in an accessible format. The Public Sector Equality Duty aims to ensure that public authorities actively consider equality when carrying out their day-to-day functions and reflect this in their policies and how they deliver their services.

NHS England is concerned that:

> *'Despite the existence of legislation and guidance, in reality many service users continue to receive information from health and social care organisations in formats which they are unable to understand and do not receive the support they need to communicate. This includes, but is not limited to, people who are blind or have some visual loss, people who are d / Deaf or have some hearing loss, people who are deafblind, and people with a learning disability. This lack of access to accessible information and communication support has significant implications for patient choice, patient safety and patient experience, as well as directly impacting upon individuals' ability to manage their own health and well-being.'*[40]

Well-being

The Patient Rights (Scotland) Act 2011 gives all patients, among other things, the right to take part in decisions about their health and well-being, and to access the information and support to do so. This may include the provision of an interpreter or a sign-language interpreter, or other communication support. Specifically the act gives patients the right to be given the information they need to make informed choices about healthcare and treatment options in a way they can understand. There is a right to be told about the care and treatment options available; what the care or treatment will involve, including the risks and benefits, and what may happen if a patient does not have it; and the right to ask for more information if they want to know more.

---

39 The Equality Act bans unfair treatment in, among other things, healthcare services. It protects people from discrimination because of nine 'protected characteristics', which include age, disability and race.

40 NHS England (2015a) *Accessible Information: Implementation Plan.* Available at: https://www.england.nhs.uk/wp-content/uploads/2015/07/access-info-imp-plan.pdf (accessed February 2017).

The act stipulates:

- NHS staff must communicate clearly and openly about care and treatment.
- NHS staff should check whether a patient has understood the information given, and whether more information is required.
- Information about medicines and possible side effects must be given in a way that patients can understand.
- Patients with a long-term condition should receive clear information about that condition in a way they can understand.
- Patients should get support to manage their condition, such as being told how and when to take medication; how to control pain; and how to access other services that could help.
- Patients should be given information about their care and treatment in a format or language that meets their needs (for example, in audio format or in a language other than English).

In 2013, the Welsh Government introduced standards (the All Wales Standards) to improve communication with patients (including children and young people) with sight loss, hearing loss, or who are deaf or deafblind. Healthcare providers in Wales must ask about patients' communication needs and record this information. Their staff must be sensitive to patients' needs and trained to communicate effectively.

In practice this means:

- Appointment letters and information must be available in accessible formats such as large print, braille[41] or audio if needed.
- British Sign Language or deafblind interpreters must be provided if requested.
- Hospitals and surgeries must be well lit and have clear signs so that it is easier for patients to find their way around.
- Loop systems (for deaf people) must be installed, and staff should know how to use them.
- Patients should be able to make and/or change appointments through a variety of methods, such as telephone, email, text messaging, text phones and websites.

Since 2016,[42] all organisations in England providing NHS or publicly funded adult social care must meet the Accessible Information Standard, which requires

---

41 Braille is a system of raised dots that people read with their fingers.

42 As a requirement of the Health and Social Care Act (2012).

materials to be clear, accurate, impartial, evidence based and up to date. It ensures that people with a disability, impairment or sensory loss (and where appropriate, carers and parents), who have information or communication needs relating to their disability, get 'accessible' information about their health and care that they can read and understand (for example in Easy Read, braille or via email) and 'communication support' if they need it (for example British Sign Language interpretation). 'Accessible' information is defined as material that can be read or received and understood by the individual or group for whom it is intended. 'Communication support' is the support needed to enable effective, accurate dialogue between a professional and a service user such that they are not put at a substantial disadvantage in comparison with those who are not disabled. This includes accessible information and communication support to enable individuals to:

■ make decisions about their health and well-being

■ make decisions and choices about their care, treatment and procedures

■ self-manage their own illness, condition or disability

■ access services appropriately and independently

■ make choices about providing or withholding consent.

Ensure you understand the duties placed upon you and your organisation, which may vary depending on the part of the UK in which you work.

You or your colleagues may have special communication needs. This chapter focuses on patients, but recognises that some of the guidance provided will apply to some staff too.

> ## Reflection
>
> Try to imagine what it is like to be thirsty and unable to ask for a cup of tea on a busy ward; or to be in pain, yet powerless to ask for analgesia. Try to recall a situation where you were unable to explain yourself – perhaps you were in a foreign country, or you had lost your voice due to an infection. How did you feel? Think of any improvements you can make to the way you communicate with people who have special needs, and do everything you can to facilitate them to communicate with you.

Hearing impairment

Around 11 million people in the UK have some form of hearing loss. The degree of impairment varies from mild age-related loss, through to the 900,000 people who are severely or profoundly deaf. Someone with hearing impairment that developed later in life will probably have a spoken language, usually English, as their first or preferred language. Some, but not all, will lipread (although that doesn't mean that they will be able to understand everything being said all of the time – unfamiliar accents and poor lighting can pose problems, for example).

People who are deaf may face barriers in accessing healthcare and healthcare information, but don't make assumptions. Someone who has a hearing impairment may be able to hear perfectly well if they are using their hearing aid, and require no special adjustment – or they might hear clearly in one room, but struggle in a different one due to poor acoustics or high levels of background noise. Someone who lost their hearing later in life might speak and read English as well as a hearing person. The golden rule is to ask people how they would like to communicate and receive information.

The useful guide *Communication Rights for People who are Deaf or Hard of Hearing*[43] states:

> *'Being deaf or hard of hearing can mean different things to different people, particularly in relation to their language and communication preferences. Even if you know whether a person who is deaf prefers to use a spoken or signed language, you may not know what communication support they prefer. Never make assumptions about the best way to communicate with someone who is deaf. Always check with the person(s) how you can best communicate with them.'*

---

43 Produced by Action on Hearing Loss (formerly The Royal National Institute for the Deaf (RNID)).

(The free guide also contains some useful healthcare case studies and is worth obtaining.)

Dos and don'ts

- Do make sure you have someone's attention before you start speaking.

- Don't look away. Face the person so they can lipread.

- Do choose a place with good lighting (to allow lipreading) and little or no background noise.

- Don't mumble. Speak clearly, using plain language, normal lip movements and facial expressions.

- Do check whether the person understands what you are saying, and, if not, try saying it in a different way – drawing it, using gestures or even miming. Point to objects to give a clue – such as a cup, if you are offering a drink.

- Don't use one-word replies. Lipreading is part guesswork, so whole sentences give contextual clues.

- Do keep your voice down, as hearing-aid users find it uncomfortable if you shout. Also, a loud voice may appear aggressive. You may also be overheard by others, which could undermine confidentiality.

Many people who are born deaf, or become deaf in early life, use sign language to communicate. The number of deaf signers who use British Sign Language (BSL)[44] as their first language is estimated at 22,000.[45] Consider learning fingerspelling or some basic BSL if you have to deal with deaf patients frequently.

Don't assume that written communication can act as an alternative way of communicating: some deaf people who use speech and lipreading may have difficulty with complex written language. Always ask about preferences.

Children and young people who are deaf may benefit from information being presented in visual formats such as illustrated comic books and storybooks.

People who are deafblind (whose combined sight and hearing impairment causes difficulties with communication, access to information and mobility) may have

---

44 BSL was officially recognised by the government as being a full, independent language in its own right in 2003. It uses hand shapes, the movement of the hands and body, facial expressions and lip patterns. It also has its own grammar, vocabulary and idioms. In Northern Ireland, Irish Sign Language (ISL) may be used.

45 Census 2011.

more complex needs. There are approximately 250,000 deafblind people in the UK. Of these, 220,000 are aged seventy or over. The degree of visual impairment and hearing loss will vary from person to person, and for the same individual across time as their hearing or sight changes. Find out how they prefer to communicate or access information.

Some patients will require communication support, such as a lipspeaker, sign-language interpreter, speech-to-text reporter, or an electronic or manual note-taker. Speak to the relevant person in your organisation about accessing these. In some situations you may have to resort to using someone who is not a registered communications support professional, in order to overcome an immediate communication barrier in the absence of a professional being available. In such circumstances, ensure that the patient is aware that the communicator is not qualified and registered, and also check that they consent to using that person – although in an emergency this may not be possible. When using a communications support professional, always look at and address the patient, not the other professional.

Finally, look out for the patient who has an unacknowledged hearing impairment. There are people who will not admit, even to themselves or their families, that they are struggling to hear. They may ask you to repeat information, speak with an especially loud (or quiet) voice, or they might misunderstand what you say. Sometimes you can see that someone is having difficulty. Amend your communication style accordingly.

Visual impairment

Around two million people in the UK have some form of sight loss, and 360,000 people are registered as blind or partially sighted. Visual impairment is where the ability to see is impaired to such a degree that it causes problems that cannot be remedied by simple means such as glasses or contact lenses. It can range from mildly impaired vision that affects normal life, through to complete loss of sight. As such, visually impaired people will have a range of different needs when it comes to communicating, depending on their level of impairment. Some will be able to:

- read information – so long as it is printed in black, minimum 14-point-size font on non-shiny white paper
- read websites and electronic documents on a computer, using magnifiers and screen readers

■ read braille – according to the RNIB (Royal National Institute for Blind People), braille is the preferred reading medium of approximately 18,000 blind and partially sighted adults in the UK.

Unless a patient is deafblind or has a profound learning disability, the majority should be able to digest information in digital audio formats such as CDs and MP3 files – although not everyone will have the knowledge or technology to play them.

The RNIB offers a range of services to other organisations, including providing detailed guidance on making information accessible to people who have sight loss. When it comes to printed information, here are some dos and don'ts:

Dos and don'ts

■ Do use a 'sans serif' font. (Fonts with decorative flourishes at the ends of the letters are serif fonts. Those without flourishes are sans serif.)

■ Don't use small print. A minimum of 14-point-size font for printed materials. (The point size for large print is 16-22.)

■ Do use Arial, Helvetica and Futura fonts, as they are easier to read.

■ Don't use capital letters for entire words or sentences. Uppercase letters are more difficult to read quickly, as the distinctive shape of words is lost and everything looks 'blocky'.

■ Do have unjustified right margins (the text is aligned with the margin on the left, but ragged on the right-hand margin).

■ Don't use large blocks of text, as they can be difficult for partially sighted people to read. Stick to shorter paragraphs if possible, and leave a space between paragraphs.

■ Do use matt-finish paper. A glossy finish can produce a glare. Also avoid thin, semi-transparent paper.

For more detailed information on printed materials, see Action for Blind People's free guide, *Making it Clear: Guidelines to producing printed material for people who are blind or partially sighted.*

When you have a meeting or consultation with a blind or partially sighted person, and it is their first visit to your clinic, ask if they would like to be guided to the consultation room. Not everyone will need help in getting around. If help is required:

- Offer your arm. The visually impaired person may grip it just above the elbow, or they may prefer to grip your shoulder.

- Walk half a step in front, using a pace that is neither too fast nor too slow.

- Tell the patient if there are any steps, and specify whether they are to ascend or descend.

- When you get to the room, put the client's hand on the back of the chair so they know where to sit down.

If the client is already in the room, they may not be aware that you are approaching or have entered. Say something so that they know – and if there's anyone with you, introduce them so the patient knows who is there. Tell the patient what you are doing or about to do: 'I'm just going to wash my hands and organise my equipment, and then I will take a look in your mouth.' Or, 'We will be at the lift in a moment, and then we will travel down to the first floor for the radiography department.' If you need to leave the room, explain: 'I just need to get the nurse to help with this. I will be back in two minutes.' Warn patients about anything that may otherwise cause alarm: 'I am about to wheel the trolley over a raised area and it might feel a bit bumpy, but don't worry – you're completely safe.'

When it comes to hospital and care home admissions, people with a more severe visual impairment may face particular challenges. Be sensitive to these. Hospital menus can be a problem if the print is too small to read. Keep a magnifier on the ward, just in case; provide a good reading light; enlarge text on a photocopier; or read information aloud where necessary. If possible, give someone a bed that is easy to find, such as the first one in the ward. Make sure they know where to find important things – the kind of things that would be obvious to a sighted person – such as where the toilets are, or the call bell. It can be very disorientating for anyone admitted to hospital, but a visual impairment can exacerbate this feeling.

When a partially sighted person is accompanied by someone, always address your questions to the patient and not their carer or relative. (Unless you do wish to involve the relative in the conversation, as co-partner in care. But even then, the primary communication should remain with the patient.)

Learning disability

Around 1.5 million people in the UK have a learning disability, meaning that they have a reduced intellectual ability and have difficulty with everyday activities such as household tasks and money management. They tend to take longer to learn and may need support to understand complicated information and interact with others. Needs will vary. People with a mild learning disability require minimal support to live an independent life (perhaps just a bit of help with form-filling, for example). Those with a severe or profound learning disability may need full time care and support with every aspect of their life.

People with a learning disability may take longer to process information, and this can be exacerbated (as it is for anyone) when in a stressful situation such as visiting a hospital. By speaking a bit more slowly, you can help someone take in what you're saying. Use shorter sentences too, and everyday language. Convey only one idea per sentence, because some people with a learning disability will focus in on key words, which may get lost in a longer, complex sentence. There is a good example of the importance of this in the *Hospital Communication Book*,[46] which can be downloaded free from the Mencap website (www.mencap.org.uk). A doctor says to a patient with a learning disability, 'Unfortunately, due to complications, it's not possible for you to go home yet; we may know more tomorrow.' The patient focuses on the words 'home' and 'tomorrow', and gets the wrong message altogether.

Dos and don'ts

- Do use appropriate gestures to reinforce your spoken message where appropriate.

- Don't use abstract phrases such as 'The consultant is doing her rounds', as this could cause confusion.

- Do find the best way to communicate. Ask family, friends or support workers, if necessary, when someone has difficulty communicating.

- Don't forget that if someone has a severe or profound learning disability, parents and carers may be able to tell you which signs and behaviours indicate distress.

Like adults, children and young people with learning disabilities will vary in their needs. Some may not be able to access information through words, pictures or diagrams and will need dedicated one-to-one communication help and support. Establish what level of support (if any) is required.

'Easy Read' is an effective method of providing accessible written information

---

46 The Learning Disability Partnership Board in Surrey. *The Hospital Communication Book*. Available at: https://www.mencap.org.uk/sites/default/files/2016-06/hospitalcommunicationbook.pdf (accessed February 2017).

to people with learning disabilities. You can find out more in Chapter 8. The language programme 'Makaton' can be useful for people with profound learning disabilities. It uses signs and symbols to support spoken language and help people to communicate. The signs and symbols – which are used with speech, in spoken word order – help provide extra clues about what someone is saying. The signs can help people who have no speech or whose speech is unclear. The symbols can help people who have limited speech or who cannot, or prefer not to, use sign language. You can find out more about Makaton at www.makaton.org.

Audio and audiovisual information (on CD, MP3 or video format) can also be useful for people with a learning disability if they find it difficult to absorb information. After a consultation, the information can be played at home, to refresh memory and understanding.

Dementia and other cognitive impairment

Cognitive impairment covers a wide spectrum. Residents or patients with a mild cognitive impairment – the kind that affects some people when they grow older, such as being a little forgetful or a bit slower at making decisions – may be able to communicate and understand perfectly well. At the other end will be residents with advanced Alzheimer's and other forms of dementia, who are unable to speak and whose cognition and memory is severely and permanently affected. Some patients will be only temporarily impaired, following mild trauma, anaesthetic, or medication that has left them drowsy or less alert. People with brain trauma or who have had a stroke may be affected temporarily or permanently. Adapt communication to meet the needs of the individual and their type and level of impairment.

The Alzheimer's Society stated that in 2016 there were 850,000 people with dementia in the UK, with one person developing the disease every three minutes. One in six people over the age of eighty have it, and over 40,000 people under sixty-five do too. Seventy percent of people in care homes have dementia or severe memory problems. More than 25,000 people from black and minority ethnic groups in the UK are affected. Given these numbers, even if you don't work in the field of dementia, you will most likely have to treat patients with the condition.

Aphasia

Aphasia is an acquired communication disorder caused by damage or injury to language parts of the brain. It can range from mild to severe. It may be found in people who have had a stroke, and it affects a person's ability to use or understand words, although intelligence is unimpaired. People may have difficulty speaking and finding the right words, and struggle to understand conversations, comprehend written words, write words, use numbers and do simple calculations. Symptoms may be exacerbated when they are tired or in noisy environments. There are many types of aphasia, each of which can affect communication in different ways.

Expressive or non-fluent aphasia

People with expressive aphasia know what they want to say, but struggle to say, write or sign it (if they previously used sign language). Speech will be slow, halting, laboured, disjointed and ungrammatical. Sentences may be pared back to essential words only, with unimportant words omitted – 'want nurse' rather than 'please can you call the nurse'. Despite this, patients may still manage to make themselves understood, although they may be very frustrated at their lack of fluency and difficulty in turning their thoughts, ideas and wishes into spoken or written words. In very severe forms, a client may only be able to manage single words, and communication will be more challenging. Although patients may have only limited difficulty in understanding what you say to them, consider keeping to simple (non-patronising) sentence structures. Such patients may be able to understand written information.

Receptive or fluent aphasia

People with receptive aphasia struggle to understand the meaning of written and spoken language, and gestures – although they retain their other cognitive abilities. They may be unable to comprehend your message, although they will be unaware that they have a disorder. They will speak fluently, using nonsensical sentences containing random or invented words. They may neglect conversational courtesies such as turn-taking or continuing to speak when most of us would pause to allow contributions from other people.

At one end of the scale, difficulties may be limited to understanding strong accents or fast speech – although the ability to carry out simple instructions is not impaired. A common symptom of receptive aphasia is taking statements literally rather than figuratively: 'The doctor will give you a bell when the test results arrive,' may leave the listener expecting a bell rather than a phone call. At the other end of the scale, patients may have severely disturbed language comprehension.

As cognitive impairments cover such a broad range of conditions and span such a wide spectrum of impairment, the usual rule applies: communicate in the most appropriate way for the individual in front of you.

Dos and don'ts

■ Do face the patient you are addressing (not their relative/carer), sit at their level and make friendly eye contact.

■ Don't start the conversation until you have their attention.

■ Do explain who you are if they don't know/remember you, and the purpose of the encounter if necessary.

■ Don't use medical jargon. Use simple language and simple sentence structures.

■ Do have conversations in quiet and distraction-free places.

■ Don't forget to switch off the TV (turning the volume down may be insufficient, as distracting images will remain on the screen).

■ Do use props to aid understanding: for example, show their coat, if suggesting a walk; or a tea cup, if offering a drink.

■ Don't use personal pronouns; use names instead: for example, Jimmy/Jimmy's rather than he/him/his.

When talking to someone who is cognitively impaired, speak more distinctly than you might usually, but don't shout or raise your voice. Remember that you're addressing an adult and don't patronise. Where you have a lot of information to impart, spread it over a number of sessions if possible to avoid the patient losing the thread of what is being said.

Break instructions into simple steps that can be more easily understood, and omit unnecessary steps. Tell patients what's going to happen, and repeat as required so that they understand, rephrasing if necessary. Use gestures to help someone understand what you are saying. If the patient can read, provide written information to support what you have said.

When it comes to asking questions, keep them specific: 'Would you like a cup of tea?' rather than 'Are you feeling thirsty just now?' Don't ask several things at once: 'Would you like tea or coffee, and do you fancy a biscuit or some toast with it?' Break multiple questions into single enquiries. Although open questions are preferable in many situations, consider asking closed yes/no questions with someone who is cognitively impaired: 'Would you like a biscuit with your tea?' rather than 'What would you like with your tea?' Use nouns rather than 'it' or 'them'. Ask 'Do you want milk in your tea?' rather than 'Do you want milk in it?'

Be patient and allow clients sufficient time to process what you have said and to respond, including time for thinking and finding the right words. Don't interrupt, but if appropriate, help out by using prompts or further questions to enable you to understand their message. Don't get into futile arguments. If a resident falsely accuses you of stealing their dentures, don't react in the same way as you would with a person who was not cognitively impaired. Instead, helpfully suggest that you help look for the missing item.

Brain injury

Headway, the brain injury association, says that damage to the right side of the brain may lead to a person interpreting verbal information literally. A common expression such as 'This will only take a minute' may cause the patient to get upset if you take longer than 60 seconds. Ability to grasp humour or sarcasm may similarly be affected. The subtle nuances of conversation may pass them by, and the result of all of this can be that things are taken the wrong way. Be alert to this possibility and careful of the way you phrase things. If something is taken the wrong way, leading to a negative reaction, don't take it personally or start getting defensive.

Social communication difficulties may arise where there has been a frontal brain injury. Verbal and non-verbal cues may be missed. For example, you may have a waiting room full of patients and give off cues that an appointment needs to end (such as looking at the clock or tidying your desk). You may need to be explicit: 'I'm sorry Mrs Smith, but we must end the consultation now, as I have other patients to see.'

Someone with a brain injury may say the wrong thing at the wrong time, talk too much about themselves, swear inappropriately, or abruptly switch to another topic. This can make such patients appear rude or insensitive. They may dominate the conversation, or not realise that it's their turn to make a contribution. Fear of forgetting their point may cause them to interrupt. All of this may impede the building of a therapeutic relationship. Remind yourself that any social difficulties are caused by the brain injury, not by the patient's wilful intent.

When caring for a moderate to severely impaired person in a hospital or residential home, be sensitive. It will be a confusing situation for the patient, and they may be scared and disorientated. You may be rushed, but don't make them feel hurried. Talk to residents about what you need to do. Don't just take off their clothes: explain that you need to put on a clean nightdress. Don't shove some pills in their mouth: explain that it's time for their medicine. Non-verbal communication can be used to great effect to provide reassurance – a friendly smile, for example. Try to be flexible and responsive. If a patient struggles when you try to get them up in the morning, perhaps you can leave it for now. Return in 10 minutes and try again, as they might be less resistant and more receptive. Don't see everything from your perspective as a series of tasks to be accomplished in a certain order or timescale. Try to understand how it feels from the resident's view, and be as flexible and amenable as possible within the constraints of a busy home or ward.

Dos and don'ts

- Do be kind, gentle and patient.

- Don't discuss the client in their presence, as if they were not there.

- Do remember that the tone of your voice can be reassuring (or alarming), so reflect on how you sound as well as what you say.

- Don't forget relatives. They may know how the client can be helped to communicate.

- Do pay attention to a client's body language, such as posture and facial expressions, which can show whether someone is in pain or discomfort.

When dealing with patients in a coma state, speak to them in the same way that you would if they were awake. Although they are unable to communicate with you, they may be able to hear and understand what you are saying. When you come into the room, announce who you are and why you are there: 'Hello Jenny, I'm the nurse on duty this afternoon. I've come to check that you …' Do not say anything in front of the patient that you would not say were they not in a coma.

Children and young people

Good communication lies at the heart of facilitating children and young people to exercise their right to be active participants in decision-making about their care and to understand their condition, any treatments and potential side effects. They can be supported in this by clear, relevant, up-to-date information – both written and oral. The level of their involvement will depend on their age and cognitive ability, but their rights must not be overlooked and should be actively promoted by healthcare professionals – even in the face of dissent by their adult parents/carers.

Give at least as much attention to what children tell you as to what their parents/ carers say. Do not assume that something should be given greater credence because an adult says it – although, of course, parents/guardians do need to be listened to respectfully. The child, as patient, probably has a better understanding or insight into how something affects them.

There are times when it is appropriate to have a parent or guardian to act as mediator or interpreter of complex messages and to provide explanations to their children and young people. However, do not rely solely on this route: the parent or guardian may not always be present. Furthermore, children and young people have a right to access healthcare information independently of their parent/carer, so you will need to ensure that you are able to provide it in a form that can be understood and that meets their needs. Children and young people, like adults, have a right to have information, and they also have a right to ask not to know something. They may not wish to know their prognosis, for example, and such wishes must be respected.

Young people with disabilities will most likely have a greater number of medical interventions and treatments than able-bodied children, and yet their scope for making decisions about this may be restricted by the often higher degree of adult intervention in their lives. When communicating with young people who have a disability, empower them to articulate their issues and concerns, wishes and preferences.

Like other groups, children and young people are not all the same. They comprise individuals with differences and varying needs. There is huge variety in cognitive ability even within the distinct age groups from toddler to child to teenager to young adult – and practitioners' communication style must reflect that variety. The cognitive ability of one thirteen-year-old, for example, may be very different to that of another teen of the same age. Most children become more independent with age, and their ability to communicate improves, but in young people with a degenerative condition it may begin to decline.

It can be difficult to get the balance right when communicating with children and young people. On the one hand, it is important not to underestimate or patronise them; on the other, if you overestimate their emotional maturity and ability to understand a complex message, you may fail to communicate effectively and appropriately. Children are able to understand concepts if they are set out in a clear and accessible way. Most can also handle distressing messages if presented honestly yet sensitively, empathetically and in a supportive way.

Reflection

Think back to your childhood and see if you can recall an adult with whom you had a good relationship. Think about how they communicated with you. Do you feel confident when it comes to communicating with children and young people? Do you speak to them directly, using appropriate body language and suitable words for their age and stage, or do you tend to address the adult in the room? How might you improve the way you deal with children and young people?

Sit at their level when discussing anything with a child or young person. Use a calm, reassuring voice when speaking. Establish how much they know about their diagnosis, condition, treatment and any alternatives, and prognosis. You will need to be able to fill in any gaps using an age-appropriate explanation and possibly visual aids too – such as books, dolls or soft toys. Timing is important, so if possible avoid imparting (or gathering) information when a child is tired, afraid or in pain. Think ahead about what information is needed and how best to deliver it. Give information in manageable chunks, allowing each piece to be absorbed and understood before moving on to the next. Remember to check that what you have said has indeed been properly understood.

Exploring emotions can be difficult, depending on the age of the young person. Think about how you can encourage children and young people to express themselves. You may choose to encourage a child to use other ways of showing how they feel, such as by drawing, painting, making a collage or creating something from clay or play-dough. Where appropriate, family members such as parents and siblings may be able to open up conversations that encourage a child or young person to start talking about feelings and emotions.

Dos and don'ts

- Do listen carefully to what children and young people say, and take it seriously.

- Don't rush. Allow sufficient time. A consultation with a child or young person may take longer.

- Do address comments and questions directly to children and young people, and only to their parents where appropriate.

- Don't forget the benefits of reinforcing spoken information with written information (including in comic-strip and storybook form) and information in other formats – such as making it available online, in audio and visual formats such as MP3 and CD.

- Do use age-appropriate language with children ('cleaning teeth' rather than 'dental hygiene'; 'poo' rather than 'stool' or 'bowel motion').

- Don't use jargon. Find out how they refer to body parts, and use those terms when speaking to children.

Producing information for young people

If producing written or visual information for children and young people, engage your organisation's communications professionals and ensure that they involve young people in shaping the content and design. Consider also consulting youth workers, teachers and others who are expert in dealing with these age groups.

The Patient Information Forum's *Guide to Producing Health Information for Children and Young People* (2014) states that Great Ormond Street Hospital and the Institute for Child Health suggest that when creating information for children and young people, separate versions should be produced for each of the following age ranges:

- *Under sevens:* storybook-style information works well with this age group in explaining information.

- *Eight-to eleven-year-olds:* this age group can ask questions to clarify meaning, give their opinions and modify them in light of new information, and make decisions. The question-and-answer format works well for them.

- *Over twelves:* young people can distinguish between fact and opinion and can understand quite complicated concepts if explained clearly. They can search for information independently online. They can make informed choices and explain the reasons for their choice. They like information to be communicated to them in the form of facts, Q&As and personal stories.

When speaking with very young children, remember that children up to the age of four utilise play to communicate, and it can be used to communicate with them too. Use dolls or teddy bears to point to areas of the body or to show a child what is happening.

True story

I took my daughter Ellie for a routine childhood vaccination. The health visitor who was giving it 'ambushed' Ellie by appearing from behind with a loaded syringe. Ellie took fright and tried to escape from the surgery, screaming. I tried to calm things and to reassure Ellie, but the damage was done, and Ellie was adamant that 'that nasty nurse' was not touching her. Establish rapport before attempting to touch a child. Chat with the child and explain what's going to happen. If it is going to hurt, be honest and say that it will hurt a little bit, 'but I can see that you're a really brave little girl'. To this day, Ellie can recall the incident – and she's now nineteen.

Communicating with non-verbal children

Just because a child can't speak, it doesn't mean that they have no opinions and nothing to say. A child might be non-verbal due to an anxiety disorder (selective mutes, for example, understand what's said but cannot respond in certain situations, even though they are able to speak) or because of a medical condition. There are many ways of communicating with such children, depending on their preferences. Some children have a 'communication passport', a simple and practical guide to help others communicate with them. It contains personal information about the child's needs, such as their medical condition, likes and dislikes. A communication passport can give the child a voice and helps others to understand them. It also provides the child with some control when it comes to communicating and indicating their choices. Passports can be very useful in helping healthcare professionals quickly to understand the child's personal needs and preferences.

Some children make choices by pointing to a symbol or word in a communication book or on a communication chart. They might use a fist or a finger, or point with their eyes or with a head pointer. Others use smartphone apps. Photos and other images on mobile phones can also be used. Children with selective mutism may communicate using gestures such as nodding or shaking their head, or they may manage to speak a word or two, often in a whisper. More information, including communications advice from parents of children with disabilities, can be found on the website of Scope, the disability charity (www.scope.org.uk).

Never use children as a communications intermediary, to act as interpreters for a parent or sibling who cannot communicate with you. It is a big burden for them, and their relative may not want to share private medical information with another family member – especially a child or young person. It's fair to no one.

People with dyslexia

Around 10% of the population has some degree of dyslexia.[47] It is well known that dyslexia affects the ability to read, write and spell (and you can read more about that in Chapter 8). But did you know that it also affects the way information is processed, stored and retrieved, memory, organisation and sequencing? People with dyslexia may have difficulty remembering and following spoken instructions, such as a medication regime or wound-care instructions, and struggle to concentrate in busy environments such as A&E because of heightened sensitivity to noise and visual stimuli. If your patient has dyslexia, establish where on the spectrum they are (from mild to severe) and what kind of support they need from you. The following advice is based on that given by the British Dyslexia Association:

---

47   Dyslexia Action (2016). Available at: http://www.dyslexiaaction.org.uk/page/about-dyslexia-0.

- Give clear, concise and direct instructions. Be specific rather than hinting.

- Give instructions one at a time: Don't say, 'Remove the old dressing and discard, then clean the wound using the antiseptic wipes provided.' Break it into individual steps: 'Remove the old dressing. Throw it away. Clean the wound. Use the …'

- Communicate instructions slowly and clearly in a quiet location.

- Demonstrate if possible, in addition to explaining using words. Allow the patient to video the demonstration on their phone if they wish.

- Write down important information. (When providing written information, follow the advice in Chapter 8, as people with dyslexia have specific requirements.)

- Encourage the patient to take notes if it will help them understand or retain the information.

- Allow the patient to use a digital recorder or their telephone to record important instructions, if they wish.

- Don't assume that you have been understood. Ask for instructions to be repeated back, to confirm that the instruction has been understood correctly: 'I've explained how to clean your wound. Can I ask you explain it back to me so I'm clear that you have understood?'

People with dyslexia usually also have 'working-memory' difficulties. Working memory holds temporary information of the type that is used to process facts and make decisions. (Working-memory difficulties can also affect many people with dyspraxia; those with ADHD; people with multiple sclerosis; stroke survivors and people with neurological trauma.) People with dyslexia may, for example, find it hard to hold several pieces of working information at the same time, while being asked questions. Clearly this can make a clinical consultation quite stressful and difficult for them. Additionally they may have short-term memory problems, and struggle when it comes to names, numbers, dates and facts. Take great care explaining numbers, as misunderstanding could lead to medication errors. Reversing numbers is not unusual, so encourage the patient to say the numbers out loud, write them down or press a calculator's buttons to check the figures have been understood. They may also have problems remembering appointments, so ask if they need a reminder. Their difficulty in presenting a sequence of events in a logical, structured way may make history-taking more difficult for you with dyslexic patients. They may have poorer listening and concentration skills, so be sure to check that they have heard and understood.

People not fluent in English

Researchers at Loughborough University – whose research investigated healthcare professionals' (physiotherapists, paramedics, doctors, nurses, pharmacists and receptionists) perceptions of caring for people from minority ethnic groups with poor or no English language skills – wrote that in healthcare there is evidence that 'language and literacy barriers adversely affect clinical effectiveness, medical decision making, medication adherence, and patients' understanding of and access to services'[48] and that 'patients with language and literacy difficulties are more likely to be hospitalised'. The researchers found that 'language barriers were the main obstacle in eliciting an accurate medical history, explaining and gaining pain scores, communicating reasons for patient transport delays, arranging appointments by telephone, explaining medication and side effects or diagnosing and communicating problems'. For these reasons, it is essential that healthcare professionals address the communications issues that affect people who are not fluent in English.

Do not make assumptions about people's proficiency in English. Never assume that anyone who is non-white is not a fluent English speaker (or that anyone who's white is fluent); don't conclude that someone with a foreign accent (or name) will be unable to speak the language proficiently; or that people dressed a certain way (wearing a hijab, sari or a turban, for example) will not understand English. The key, always, is to regard everyone as an individual. Establish their understanding at the outset and make any necessary adjustments. You may find that some people born and brought up in the UK also struggle to understand some of what you say.

A study[49] by emergency medicine researchers of 700 adults in England showed that between 46.5% and 87% (depending on the question posed) did not have a correct understanding of the meaning of the word 'unconscious' – even though many of them believed that they knew what it meant. All could speak English, although not all were native speakers of the language.

Unsurprisingly, comprehension of the term was significantly poorer among those for whom English was not their first language: 62.7% as opposed to 77.8% for native English speakers. However, this research demonstrates that even terms that might be regarded as non-technical, that are used in everyday parlance,

---

48 Taylor SP, Nicolle C & Maguire M (2013) Cross-cultural communication barriers in health care. *Nursing Standard* **27** (31) 35–43.

49 Cooke NW, Wilson S, Cox P & Roalfe A (2000) Public understanding of medical terminology: non-English speakers may not receive optimal care. *Journal of Accident and Emergency Medicine* **17** 119–121.

can in fact be widely misunderstood by significant numbers of native English speakers too – in the case of this study, almost a quarter.

The researchers concluded:

'Those who do not have English as their first language may receive a lower priority of ambulance response because of their misunderstanding of a common medical term. In the A&E department they may be triaged for a longer wait, not receive necessary radiography, or fail to be admitted for observation because their misunderstanding results in them stating a person was not unconscious. Alternatively they may be over investigated and over-utilise resources because of misunderstanding that labels someone unconscious when they are not.'

This study showed that there was real value in asking supplementary questions in order to elicit the correct answer. In the case of establishing whether someone was or had been unconscious, supplementary questions may include asking whether the patient was standing up or talking – or more generically, asking how they were behaving. Also consider asking what the patient understands by a particular term, so you can establish their level of comprehension and have confidence in the reliability of any answers. Consider any additional clarifying questions that you can ask, so you are sure that you have the correct information on the condition of your patient.

When speaking to people whose first language is not English, you may have to make adjustments to how you speak if they are not fluent. Do so in a way that is not patronising or offensive – such people are not stupid! Indeed, those who are able to master more than one language may well be smarter in certain ways. An article on the British Council's website states that bilingualism affects the brain in a number of positive ways:

'These skills make up the brain's executive control system, which looks after high-level thought, multi-tasking, and sustained attention. Because bilingual people are used to switching between their two languages, they are also better at switching between tasks, even if these tasks are nothing to do with language.' [50]

When speaking to someone who is not very proficient in English, remember that everyone is an individual and levels of comprehension will vary. Tailor your response accordingly. Healthcare receptionists interviewed as part of a research

50 Muñoz MA (2014) *Does Bilingual Make you Smarter?* Available at: https://www.britishcouncil.org/voices-magazine/does-being-bilingual-make-you-smarter (accessed February 2017).

study[51] said that some patients with poor or no English language skills made excuses about filling forms in outpatient clinics. Nurses had to be called to help. The receptionists agreed that were patients to be sent forms with questions about their condition with their appointment letters, this could help avert problems with form filling in the clinic, as it would give patients more time to get assistance to complete forms. Do you do this in your workplace?

In the same study, receptionists reported fear and anxiety among patients about finding various departments, particularly when outside the main hospital building. Do you provide signage in the main languages spoken in the communities you serve – or even just in plain English (*Heart Department* rather than *Cardiology*; *X-Ray Department* rather than *Radiology*), or multilingual medicine labels and hospital menus?

Dos and don'ts

- Do pronounce words clearly.

- Don't use idioms and colloquial terms (such as 'Are you feeling blue?' or 'I'll drop you a line/give you a bell about your next appointment'), as they may not be understood. Such expressions' literal meaning is very different from what is intended.

- Do use shorter, less complex sentences.

- Don't use long, less familiar words. It's better to use several shorter ones instead.

- Don't use jargon and technical terms if possible.

- Do slow the pace of your speech to allow your patient to keep up.

- Don't raise your voice: speak at normal volume.

- Do pay particular attention if you have a strong accent, or speak in a dialect – reflect on whether you will need to modify how you speak in order to be understood.

- Do consider asking supplementary clarifying questions to reassure you that your patient really understands you.

It is easy to cause confusion when speaking to someone who is less familiar with English. Look out for expressions that may be ambiguous. For example, a patient suffering from anxiety is asked: 'How did you find coming to the clinic today?' The clinician is trying to establish how stressful the journey was, but

---

51 Taylor SP, Nicolle C & Maguire M (2013) Cross-cultural communication barriers in health care. *Nursing Standard* **27** (31) 35–43.

the patient thinks they're being asked whether they were able to find the clinic. A more direct 'How stressful was your journey to the clinic today?' would avert misunderstanding.

When writing information for people whose first language is not English, the advice in Chapter 8 on plain English should be applied. Information written in plain language is easier for everyone, regardless of level of education, nationality or age. Plain English is also easier to translate into other languages – and to subtitle, in the case of videos for people with a hearing impairment. If you do translate information, consider 'back translation', where someone fluent in both languages translates it back into English. Such an exercise will highlight any potential translation problems.

Where patients speak little or no English, finding a translator may be necessary. Beware using a family member as it could compromise a patient's privacy, and they (or the relative) might be embarrassed at having to discuss/pass on sensitive medical matters. There is also a risk that a relative may censor or put their own spin on what is being said by the patient or the practitioner. Use a professional, independent interpreter. Remember to address the patient, not the interpreter. Patients may sometimes misunderstand the role of the interpreter. Researchers speaking to physiotherapists found that there are times when the patient, when presented with a choice of treatments, asks the interpreter what they would suggest. It is for you to explain at the outset the role of the interpreter so as to avert misunderstanding. You will need more time for a consultation involving an interpreter, so be sure to schedule a sufficiently long slot.

Chapter 6: Communicating in difficult or challenging situations

Healthcare professionals can find themselves in challenging situations that need to be managed with special care. This could involve having to deal with people who are aggressive, angry, abusive, hostile or confrontational; people who are 'difficult' or uncooperative; and those who refuse reasonable requests. This chapter shows how to manage – and even avert – potentially tricky situations using practical techniques.

When you decided to become a healthcare professional, you no doubt realised that it was not going to be an easy career choice, but there can be days when it can all feel just too hard. Sometimes a number of factors come together to create a situation that can drain you of warmth and compassion. You might be struggling with problems at home, while at work you're stressed with an over-large caseload, you've missed your lunch break for the third day in a row, your line manager is complaining about you – and then you're faced with an unpleasant patient, or there's another abusive drunk in A&E. Days like that can be challenging, but simple communications techniques can help you cope.

Healthcare practitioners are taught to be non-judgemental, so labelling the individual as unpleasant may be unhelpful. It is better to think of the interaction as difficult rather than the patient. Writing for the BMJ Careers website, Marika Davies, of the Medical Protection Society in London, says that it is widely recognised that the factors that contribute to a difficult situation can be broadly grouped into four categories: patient, doctor, disease, and system.

- **Patients:** Some clients make unreasonable demands, or can be disruptive. Others may be pleasant, but are nevertheless difficult to deal with because of their unrealistic expectations, their refusal to take responsibility for their health and well-being, or for the fact that they are the 'worried well'. Others are quite simply disagreeable, manipulative or whiney. Some patients are more likeable than others. This is fine so long as you do not let that show in your demeanour or in the care that you provide.

- **Healthcare professionals:** Practitioners sometimes contribute to making the interaction difficult if feeling low due to stress, worry, hunger, tiredness, headaches, or other factors. Professionals are human beings who may react badly to a patient or a patient's attitudes, and feel angry or resentful. However, that's no excuse for letting negative feelings show, or providing suboptimal care.

- **Disease:** Problems may arise due to patients' natural stress and anxiety about the situation; illicit drug or alcohol use; the side effects of prescribed medications on mood; or certain medical conditions.

- **System:** The NHS, not-for-profit, and even private sectors are under financial pressure, which affects availability of resources and places health and social care professionals under increased pressure. This adds to the difficulties faced day-to-day.

It is helpful to recognise the factors that are at work – including your own emotional reactions – and to understand how they can combine to create a situation that may be challenging to manage. The more factors there are, the greater the challenge will be. Nevertheless, as a professional it is incumbent upon you to take control of a potentially difficult situation and to de-escalate or otherwise defuse it, making for a more positive encounter for patient and practitioner alike. You don't want to feel tense, angry or frustrated, do you? By approaching potentially difficult interactions in a positive way, you can often emerge from them feeling more upbeat and satisfied. That will in turn create a stronger patient/professional therapeutic relationship. I have heard anecdotes about particularly cantankerous patients who have reacted incredibly positively to small kindnesses, such as a smile and a cup of tea. Sometimes simply knowing that someone cares can bring a turnabout in attitude.

No healthcare staff should be subjected to violence, assault or obscenities, but regrettably anger, aggression and hostility in the form of verbal abuse and threatening behaviour can sometimes go with the territory, particularly for those working in mental health and A&E – and it often goes unreported too. Poor communication has been found to be a trigger in certain cases. Another background factor is that many healthcare encounters are highly emotionally charged, involving a lot of fear and worry, pain and distress – for the patient and their friends and relatives.

It is a normal human reaction to take hostility personally and to feel that it is directed at you as an individual. This may not be the case. Patients and their relatives may be facing stresses and pressures that will most likely not bring out the best in them, so try to understand the underlying cause of their behaviour. By putting yourself in their shoes, and showing care, compassion and empathy, you may be able to win people round and secure their co-operation. It can be challenging to show warm reactions to people who are displaying anger or aggression, when all you are trying to do is help them, but staying in control of your own emotions is vital.

In dealing with this kind of behaviour, it can be helpful to identify and try to understand the causes. These might include:

- **Bad news:** If a patient or relative has been told of a death or a devastating diagnosis, their reaction may be easier to understand.

- **Intoxication:** Alcohol and drugs can alter normal behaviour, decrease inhibitions and make individuals more aggressive.

- **Some head injuries:** The frontal lobes are the part of the brain where reason and emotion interact. Damage to them can impair judgement, and result in personality changes including inappropriate conduct and aggressive outbursts.

- **Certain psychiatric conditions:** Such patients may be confused, have impaired ability to deal with frustration, or suffer other emotional instability.

- **Pain:** This raises stress levels and can lead to short tempers.

- **Frustration:** Long waits in A&E, for example, can make people who are tense and in pain react inappropriately. Equally, being asked the same questions by different parts of the system can be frustrating – first the NHS 111/NHS 24 service, then the paramedics, the triage nurse at A&E, the doctor … it's enough for even the most patient of patients to become cross.

- **Power:** Sometimes aggression is a means of asserting power, which can show itself when someone feels under threat. Healthcare staff have the power to give and withhold treatment, which could result in a power struggle.

- **Staff attitude:** Some of your colleagues may have an attitude problem. A patient who has been upset by a staff member with an inappropriate attitude may try to take out their frustration on you.

- **Negligence:** A patient or relative may feel that the healthcare system, or the part of it that you work in, or you or one of your colleagues, have let them down, misdiagnosed, made a medical error, or are in some other way at fault.

Over and above these, there are service users who are detained under the Mental Health Act (1983) or brought into healthcare while in the custody of the police, and this loss of liberty may well also provoke aggression.

Preventing difficulties

Prevention is better than treatment, so if you can avert difficult situations from occurring, so much the better. Good communication is a key way to help avoid challenging situations from developing. Accident and emergency departments are a place where circumstances typically conspire to create difficult situations – long waits to see a doctor; people under the influence of alcohol or drugs; individuals in pain; patients in distress, and so on. It can be a perfect storm. However, research has shown that good communication can have a beneficial impact even here. After being triaged, patients appreciate updates on likely waiting times and value reassurance about their condition: 'I'm really sorry that you're having to wait so long, Mr Jones. Friday is such a busy night in here, and your wait is likely to be another three hours, although I will keep you updated as it could change depending on who else is brought in. The nurse has seen you and judged that you won't come to any harm having to wait that long, so please try to relax. There's a water fountain over there if you're feeling thirsty.' Keeping information channels open and friendly can help avert problems from developing.

On wards, see if you can 'connect' with a difficult patient by finding common ground – get to know them a bit better. Ask a few questions about them – their family, work or interests. By chatting, you can sometimes uncover an underlying concern. The patient who is angry about a long wait in A&E may actually be really worried about what's wrong with them. Anxiety can manifest in many different ways. A friendly and reassuring chat may prevent an angry person from becoming an aggressive one.

Identify at an early stage situations that may escalate, and intervene to try to dissipate tensions. Warning signs of irritated or agitated behaviour could include:

- raised voices and/or sarcastic remarks

- body language – prolonged, aggressive eye contact; invading personal space; posture such as clenched fists, a jutting chin or puffed out chest; threatening gestures such as finger pointing or foot stamping; pacing back and forth

- aggressive behaviour – patients kicking furniture or hitting themselves.

If patients are known to you – perhaps because they are inpatients on a psychiatric ward – learn about the trigger factors that can result in violence and aggression for particular individuals. You can then work to avoid these triggers.

Sometimes simple environmental factors can be used to help avert aggression. Having entertaining distractions such as music, a television or radio, books and magazines, crosswords and puzzles can relieve tension in places such as A&E or doctors surgeries. Comfortable seating, and enough seats that no one has to stand, also helps keep people calm. A water fountain, coffee machine or vending machine for drinks and snacks during long waits will at least remove hunger and thirst as sources of complaint. Calming colour schemes and non-institutional décor can play their part too.

How to de-escalate

If you encounter difficult situations as part of your work, ensure that your employers have provided training in techniques to help you avert and manage likely scenarios – including, if applicable, dealing with aggression and violence. The advice offered here relates to communications aspects, but dealing with violence may involve using restraint, which is beyond the remit of this book.

When in a threatening situation, you must consider the safety of yourself, colleagues and other patients and relatives, and also the aggressor. Assess the risks and deal with the situation yourself only if it is safe to do so. Staff such as paramedics, who are called to violent situations such as street fights or violence in public houses, should have been trained in risk assessment and should follow local protocols.

An effective way to approach de-escalating a difficult encounter is to employ all of the communications strategies outlined in this book, because good communication is one of the first things to be abandoned in a challenging situation. We tend to stop listening to people we find challenging; our interruption rate increases; our body language can become closed and even hostile; we may become defensive; and we can sometimes become argumentative or difficult ourselves. The result?

The patient becomes even more hostile, and a downward spiral begins. Direct confrontation is likely to make an already difficult situation much worse.

When you can see things going wrong, take control of the situation – but ensure you do so in a non-authoritarian way (as you don't want to make matters worse!). Do what you can to stabilise matters and to help the angry or upset person to regain control. Someone who is backed into a corner will lash out, so offer choices or a way out if possible. You may feel angry or personally affronted, but don't be provocative as it will only make matters worse – and it's unprofessional.

Don't try to speak while someone is shouting, as it is futile and may exacerbate matters. Remain calm, listen attentively and wait until they stop. Never shout back. Aside from being unprofessional, it's a smart technique not to. It's easy to shout at someone who is shouting at you; it's much harder to continue shouting at someone who is calm and respectful. Eventually the shouting patient or relative will run out of steam, allowing you an opportunity to intervene positively.

Acknowledge that the patient/relative is angry or upset: 'I can see that you're really unhappy about this.' Ask them to explain why they feel like that: 'Could you explain to me what has caused you to feel this way, please?' Listen actively and respectfully to the response, without interruption – even if it is full of sarcastic, untrue or unhelpful remarks (failure to challenge them at this point does not mean that you concur).

Show open and friendly body language such as smiling (if appropriate) and making eye contact. Take care to get the eye contact right, as too much could be interpreted as staring, which is considered an aggressive behaviour. Be sure to respect their personal space too, as an invasion could be seen as a threatening act. Also, it's safer for you to maintain a physical distance.

If you know it, consider using the person's name. This can sometimes help to defuse a situation. But take care, as what to some may be interpreted as a friendly gesture to others could appear not to be genuine. It may even be seen as patronising, so use your judgement according to the circumstances.

Keep calm and remain composed, taking care not to take any anger or insults personally. Unless you or others are in physical danger, do not make threats to call security/the police or to have them removed from the premises. At the very least, this should help to prevent the situation from degenerating. You might even turn it around and create a positive encounter.

Typical example

Bad outcome

A very angry Mrs McSween comes storming into the nursing station demanding, 'What the hell have you done to my mother?' Her elderly mother, Gladys, who is sleeping, has a large gash on her head following a slip on the ward. The nurse on duty, Sister Jones, is immediately on the defensive, and this shows in her attitude – both body language and tone of voice. She's tired and wants to go home after a long and stressful shift. What's more, Sister Jones has been taking very special care of Gladys following her fall. She feels that Mrs McSween has a cheek barging into the nursing station with that attitude. The two women clash, and Mrs McSween ends up making a complaint about her mother's fall and about Sister Jones's attitude.

Good outcome

Although Sister Jones is tired, she is able to put herself into Mrs McSween's position and to understand her reaction. She does not take the anger personally and remains calm, polite, respectful and professional. Sister Jones invites Mrs McSween to sit down, acknowledges her understandable distress and explains that she had telephoned her several times to inform her of her mother's slip but received no answer. She explains the circumstances that led to Gladys's fall and the treatment provided. She reassures Mrs McSween that her mother has been seen by the doctor and will be fine. Her injury looks worse than it actually is. She offers to bring Mrs McSween a cup of tea while she sits with her mother and asks if she would like to speak with the doctor.

A handy tactic is to articulate the disagreement: 'We seem to have rather different ideas as to treatment. Perhaps we can explore some of the alternatives, and their pros and cons, together?' This can be a useful technique for getting the area of disagreement into the open without assigning blame or criticism. A neutral statement of fact can help you both to focus on how to move forward together towards a solution or mutually acceptable outcome.

Consistent non-punitive boundary-setting can also be helpful for addressing unacceptable behaviour: 'Whenever a patient is late for an appointment three times in a row, we …' This tactic can be useful in depersonalising an action, while at the same time being firm about its unacceptability. If the same rule is applied to all patients in the same circumstances, there is a consistency and fairness about it that can be harder to challenge. Ensure that you say what is and what is not acceptable, and explain the consequences of breaches.

Never stereotype a whole group of people because of the poor behaviour of one individual. An older, male amputee who behaves badly is merely a badly behaved person; there is no justification in treating all older male amputees as if they are about to behave in that way too. Respect people as individuals and do not let experiences with one person colour your interactions with others.

Sometimes you need to recognise that you may not be best placed to deal with a situation for whatever reason. In such circumstances, consider whether a colleague may be better suited. Don't be afraid to ask for help when you need to. It could end up being better for you and better for the patient than struggling on and getting more tired or frustrated.

Dos and don'ts

- Do recognise that it's OK to have feelings yourself.
- Don't let your feelings make you act unprofessionally.
- Do always remain calm, neutral and respectful.
- Don't lose your temper, raise your voice, become angry, provocative or attempt to humiliate the aggressor.
- Do try to see it from the patient's perspective.
- Don't react; stop and think first.
- Do take a deep breath and try to relax.
- Don't let a bad experience with one patient affect your whole day/shift or your family life.
- Do say 'No' to unreasonable demands, but be prepared to manage any adverse reaction.

Zero tolerance?

I am not a healthcare professional, and have never been on the receiving end of the kind of situations that you have to deal with. However, I have observed at close quarters violent and aggressive circumstances when doing shifts with the police and the ambulance service, as a non-executive director. This experience has given me huge respect for the many dedicated staff who undertake challenging and difficult work in healthcare and the emergency services. No one should have to tolerate violence, but do zero tolerance policies blur the dividing line between abrasive and abusive behaviour? Do they leave staff over-sensitised to behaviour that people in other professions have to deal with – such as rude, unpleasant people? It is something that is worthy of some discussion and reflection.

Reflection

In many walks of life, staff must deal with bad-mannered, unlikable individuals – pub landlords/landladies, shop assistants, traffic wardens all have to deal with hostile people. It can be a daily part of all too many jobs. When someone is disagreeable, or says something nasty, does it automatically mean that they have crossed the threshold that results in the withdrawal of service? Where is that line drawn, and by whom? What is acceptable and what is not? Are insults acceptable so long as they are not racist/sexist/homophobic, or are all insults unacceptable? What do your workplace policies say on the subject? What factors should be considered? Should you take into account the fact that a patient is distressed? Does person-centredness have a place? What about the personal resilience (or lack of it) of the member of staff? Does the workplace situation make a difference? Should a prison nurse have a higher threshold for bad language directed at him/her than a nurse working on a children's ward? These are difficult questions. Reflect upon them and discuss with colleagues.

When it all gets too much

It is human to feel affected by a negative working environment – or even by a single challenging incident at work. If your feelings are affecting you adversely and persistently, talk to someone such as a colleague or your supervisor, occupational health staff, or friends/family (taking care not to breach patient confidentiality). Talking can help, and is preferable to bottling up unexpressed emotions. If you have to face difficult situations frequently, explore coping mechanisms to help you get through them – such as meditation, mindfulness or yoga.

Reflection

There can be difficult patients, there can be difficult situations, and there can be difficult healthcare professionals. Can you sometimes be difficult to deal with? Never? Really? Reflect on your own behaviour and on how colleagues and patients would describe you. What kinds of triggers or occasions make for a difficult encounter with you?

If you would like to know more about defusing difficult situations in mental health, the National Institute for Health and Care Excellence (NICE) published evidence-based guidelines in 2015 called *Violence and Aggression: Short-term management in mental health, health and community settings*, which contains much helpful advice and information about managing patients with mental health difficulties (www.nice.org.uk/guidance).

Chapter 7: Communicating bad, sad or difficult news

It is never pleasant to be the bearer of bad news, but for patients or relatives on the receiving end, it can be devastating. That's why it's so important to know the right way to break bad news, so you don't add to their distress. This chapter's practical advice will help healthcare staff to give bad, sad or difficult news with care, compassion and sensitivity.

If you've not had to do it yet, breaking bad news will be one of the hardest things you face as a healthcare practitioner. 'Bad news' is defined as bad, sad or significant information that adversely alters someone's expectations or perceptions of their present or future. It might involve the following: telling a patient that they have a terminal illness; informing a relative of a sudden and unexpected death; breaking the news to a parent that their child has a life-limiting condition; or explaining to a client that they have a long-term chronic condition that will not improve. In breaking such news, you are giving someone something unwelcome. That will always be a difficult thing to have to do.

What constitutes bad news to one person may not be perceived in the same way by another, as Clare Warnock, a practice development sister in specialist cancer services points out:

> *'Informing patients that they are to have an operation could be perceived positively by one person, as it is confirmation of a plan for life-saving or symptom-improving treatment. However, a person who has an overwhelming fear of hospitals or anaesthesia may view the news negatively.'*[52]

---

52 Warnock C (2014) Breaking bad news: issues relating to nursing practice. *Nursing Standard* **28** (45) 51–58.

The news of a death is almost always seen as bad by relatives, but sometimes there can be a sense of relief too. When my mother died, I was relieved that her terrible suffering had finally ended and she could be at peace.

Depending on your specialism, breaking bad news may be something that you are called upon to do quite frequently – or it could be a rarity. If it is a part of your work, it is important that you are good at it because so much rests on how you deliver that news. However much you care, you can exacerbate a patient's/family's distress if your delivery is awkward, cold or impersonal.

Compassion is much talked about in healthcare, and if there is a place where that compassion must come to the fore, it is when having to break bad news. Some practitioners are naturals at this, and can deliver bad news confidently yet warmly and empathetically; others, even quite senior people, may be less accomplished. Practitioners who qualified more recently may have been taught how to do it; less recently qualified staff have possibly had to learn on the job.

The way you tackle the responsibility of delivering bad news will depend on many factors, such as how well, if at all, you know the person you have to break the news to; how bad the news is and whether there are good elements (such as possible treatments/cure); and whether the news was expected by the individual or has come out of the blue.

An article in *Nursing Times*[53] said that when it comes to communicating news of a death: 'To facilitate a normal grieving process, it is essential that relatives receive excellent communication and support from healthcare professionals.' The authors (citing Harrahill[54] and McCulloch[55]) tell us: 'The way in which news is given will always be remembered by the bereaved, whether delivered well or not.' This emphasises the huge responsibility placed on healthcare staff when delivering bad news. You will leave an enduring impression, so get it right.

The first consideration is whether you are the best messenger. Do you know the patient or relatives? Would the news be best coming from someone who does? (At the very least, can you be accompanied by someone who already knows the patient/relative?) In some healthcare settings, a doctor gives news of death even where the nurse has been the primary carer, in the false belief that seniority is a consideration for relatives. The limited research in this area suggests that this is not a factor for the majority of families. Other research backs this finding,

---

53 Reid M, McDowell J & Hoskins R (2011) Breaking news of death to relatives. *Nursing Times* **107** (5) 12–15.

54 Harrahill M (2005) Giving bad news gracefully. *Journal of Emergency Nursing* **31** (3) 312–314.

55 McCulloch P (2004) The patient experience of receiving bad news from health professionals. *Professional Nurse* **19** (5) 276–280.

suggesting that the person breaking news of a bereavement should be the individual that relatives will feel most comfortable with, preferably someone known to them already.

Prepare yourself for the encounter by having the relevant information to hand; by preparing mentally to cope with the high emotions that may be displayed; and by thinking about what you will say and how you will say it – including the vocabulary that you will use.

Create the right setting – one that is private, so there will be no interruptions; comfortable (in terms of seating, lighting, temperature and decor); quiet and calm; one where there are no barriers if possible, such as a big desk between you and the patient/relative. In the case of bereavement, a non-clinical room is best, which the relatives can remain in afterwards as they may be very distressed and need space to take in the news and to compose themselves.

It is essential to open the conversation in the correct way, setting the right tone from the outset; otherwise it may be hard to get things back on track and to establish rapport. When opening the discussion, above all remember that you are dealing with real human beings who are about to be given devastating information. You are not simply a messenger, there to hand across some technical medical information. Remember your humanity, but at the same time be careful not to get emotional or involved. You work in the caring professions, so be caring and professional.

Before beginning a conversation, think about the background to it. There may be a difference between how things will play out, depending on the situation. Take the following two examples:

■ A doctor has to tell Jenny that she has terminal cancer. He has known Jenny for some months, and there have been a number of consultations. She has seen various specialists, had exploratory tests and already fears the worst.

■ Vic is admitted into hospital following a car accident. He is dead on arrival. His pregnant wife, Jean, rushes to the hospital wanting to know if her husband is OK.

In the first scenario, there is already some common ground. Doctor and patient have met previously, and the patient has some knowledge of her condition. She started the long and worrying journey months ago. In the second scenario, this is an out-of-the-blue event for which Jean is not at all prepared. Her life has been turned upside down in the space of a single day. The distress for both may be equal, but their situations are different, and it can be helpful to reflect on this and to recognise that each person is an individual with a life, friends, family, possibly work and commitments creating a unique scenario.

The breaking of bad news is often a process rather than a one-off event. Someone admitted following a fall from a ladder might be given the devastating news that they have a spinal injury, but during the course of their time in hospital, the full implications of their accident will begin to crystallise. Further questions will be asked – 'Will I ever walk again?' or 'Will I be able to have sex?' – and the answers practitioners give may constitute additional pieces of bad news. Similarly with a cancer diagnosis, the patient journey may involve a series of tests, operations and treatments in which the full seriousness of the illness unfolds stage by stage. From informing the patient of possible cancer, to finally breaking the news that it is no longer responding to treatment or that it has spread, there are many bad-news episodes along the way.

True story

I received a call from my mother's nursing home, some 250 miles away, to say that my mother was 'very poorly'. She had Alzheimer's and had been in a poorly state for over two years. I knew that she was on a downward progression, but I didn't understand what the nurse meant by 'poorly'. I asked her to elaborate, but she simply repeated that my mother was very poorly. In the end, I was the one who had to ask, 'Is my mother at the end of her life?' I found this a very difficult thing to have to say out loud, and I struggled to find the words and to maintain my composure. I couldn't bring myself to use the word 'dying' or 'close to death'. It would have helped me so much if the nurse had been clear and unambiguous in what she was telling me, sparing me the pain of having to find the words to ask that difficult question. I needed to know whether I should drop everything and drive south to be with my mother, or wait until the planned visit the following week. 'Very poorly' was too unspecific, and the lack of specificity caused me needless distress.

Most advice on how to break bad news follows a similar format. There are various guides – ABCDE, BREAKS and, perhaps the best known, SPIKES (Setting, Perception, Invitation, Knowledge, Empathy, Strategy and Summary), an acronym coined by Baile *et al* (2000) for their six-step protocol for delivering bad news. The following bullet points combine advice from various sources, including SPIKES, on how to tackle this difficult task:

- Encourage the patient to bring a friend or family member if they wish to, as this can be a valuable source of support for them.

- Welcome the patient/relative: Get the encounter off on a good footing with a genuine and warm welcome that makes everyone feel more at ease. However, you are about to deliver bad news, so don't raise false hope by an inappropriately cheerful demeanour. (If possible, try to prepare the patient/relative in advance of any pre-planned discussion that they will receive significant news.)

- Body language: Remember appropriate body language such as maintaining eye contact and using open gestures.

- Seating: Sit close if possible, without invading personal space. Bring yourself to the same level as the patient, especially if they are in bed.

- Timing: Make sure you have sufficient time so that the consultation is unrushed and there is ample opportunity for questions and explanations. Wherever possible, select a time that is convenient for the recipient of the bad news.

- Establish how much the patient knows or suspects already by asking questions such as 'Can I ask what you have been told already about your illness?'

- Listen carefully as the patient recounts what they know. Note their level of understanding, any misunderstandings or denials, and the kind of terminology they use. Also pay attention to their mood – do they seem tearful, for example?

- Establish the patient's appetite for learning the full detail of their condition and prognosis. There can sometimes be an unspoken conspiracy between a patient and practitioner in which the patient indicates, not necessarily overtly, that they do not wish to know everything. Finding out what the patient wants to know takes great sensitivity, so listen carefully and read the body language too, as it's often what is unsaid that can be most telling. (Views can change – so the patient who initially wanted the bare minimum of information may at a later stage wish to know more.)

- Give bite-sized (small) chunks of information using appropriate language and clear explanations. Don't use jargon. If possible, use the language they used earlier when recounting what they know. Avoid euphemisms such as 'growth' (say 'cancer') or 'passed away' (say 'died').

- Check as you go to ensure that they have understood what you have said, before moving on. Don't overwhelm patients with too much info in one go. They have a lot to deal with. Go at their pace.

- Allow the patient or relative to talk about how they are feeling. They may well be emotional, so consider how you will deal with any anger, grief or crying. Show appropriate care and empathy, but keep your own emotions in check.

- Don't be afraid of silences. People may need time for the message to sink in, or space to think or reflect on what they have heard.

- The encounter will need to be brought to a close, if it does not reach one naturally. Think about how this will happen, which should involve a summary of your discussion; an opportunity to ask any further questions; and clarity about what happens next (a consultation; further tests; treatment; a chance to see the body of a loved one; the issuing of a death certificate etc.).

- If it is appropriate, provide written information for patients or relatives to take away with them (for example, a leaflet on how to arrange a funeral, or a list of Q&As on a particular type of cancer).

- If appropriate, suggest sources of pastoral, spiritual or religious care – such as putting patients/relatives in touch with a hospital chaplain, local mosque/ synagogue/temple/church (see *NHS Chaplaincy Guidelines 2015: Promoting excellence in pastoral, spiritual and religious care* for further information).[56]

- Make sure, metaphorically speaking, that the door is left open (if that is appropriate) so that the patient can get in touch with you about further questions or information (or signpost them to alternative resources if appropriate).

Death and dying

In the case of sudden and unexpected deaths, there are some specific factors to consider:

- Relatives are very likely to be in a state of shock and unable to take it all in, so be prepared to repeat what you know.

- You may not know the full facts – perhaps if the death was the result of an accident or the patient was brought in as an emergency admission. Do not speculate. Stick to what you know.

- Some relatives might push you to reveal every last detail; others might want to be on their own to digest the devastating news. Be led by what they seem to want.

- In busy situations such as A&E, you might feel that spending time with relatives is wasted time, because there are patients who desperately need your help. Remember your humanity, but also be prepared to refer relatives to sources of help.

Some practitioners feel uncomfortable using words such as 'dead' and 'died' with relatives, preferring euphemistic phrases – 'he passed away', 'she's gone', 'we lost her' or 'he's given up his fight'. Be direct, so there is no confusion: 'I am so sorry,

---

56 NHS England (2015b) *NHS Chaplaincy Guidelines 2015: Promoting excellence in pastoral, spiritual and religious care*. Available at: https://www.england.nhs.uk/wp-content/uploads/2015/03/ nhs-chaplaincy-guidelines-2015.pdf (accessed February 2017).

but your father has died.' You may need to say it more than once, to reinforce a message that relatives may not want to hear.

Some people will want to know how their loved one died; others simply that they are dead. Let the relative give a steer on how much they want to know. Break the news, adding that the death was peaceful, if this was the case. That will be a comfort to relatives. Ask if there is anything more you can tell them, so there is an opportunity to ask for further detail. If people ask for further information, you may wish to say what their condition was, what treatment or symptom relief was given and so on. Do not offer distressing details, but provide honest but sensitively worded information if asked specifically.

Does your organisation have information on practical matters such as when and where to collect the death certificate, how to register the death, how to organise a funeral, or coping with bereavement? It is useful to have such material to hand, should it be required by the family. Relatives will have a lot to digest and will likely be in an emotional state, so having information they can take away and read later will be appreciated.

Invite relatives to spend time with their loved ones if they wish to, explaining that it is an opportunity to say goodbye. Don't refer to loved ones as 'the body' or 'the deceased' or use other impersonal terms.

Informing of deaths over the phone

It is preferable that bad news is delivered face-to-face, but there are circumstances where there is no alternative but to use the telephone. You may have to call someone to ask them to come to the hospital or nursing home because a relative is dead or dying. Such a call may be challenging because there are so many factors to consider.

- Establish that you are talking to the correct person.

- When calling a mobile number, check that the recipient is in an appropriate place to receive the call (such as at home, and not at the supermarket or driving a vehicle). If necessary, arrange to call back when they have parked the car or returned home.

- Listening is more important than ever, as you will not have non-verbal cues to help you judge reactions.

Often you will make a call in order to invite a relative to attend the hospital/home to receive the bad news face-to-face. They may well react by asking you the direct question you'll be dreading: 'Is my brother/wife/father dead?' Answer direct questions honestly. If relatives live a considerable distance from the hospital, there may be benefits in giving news of a death over the telephone. This will prevent a needless rush to the hospital in the vain hope of getting there in time to say goodbye. You will have to be the judge according to the circumstances.

Reflection

Have you 'lost' someone close to you – through death or divorce, for example, or been given other devastating news? How did it feel? How did you find out? What can you remember about being told? What can you learn from your own experience that can inform how you approach breaking bad news to others?

The five stages of grief

Swiss psychiatrist Elisabeth Kübler-Ross wrote a groundbreaking book in 1969, *On Death and Dying*, inspired by her work with terminally ill patients. She suggested that following a terminal diagnosis or death, the patient or close relatives experience a series of emotions: denial ('The diagnosis must be wrong'); anger ('Why me?'); bargaining ('Surely if I lose weight or give up smoking, I can get better?'); depression ('I don't want to see any visitors. What's the point?'); and acceptance ('I'd better start getting my affairs in order'). She later clarified that the five stages are not linear – anger may not follow denial, for example. They may occur in any order, not all stages will necessarily be experienced by all patients, and people may move back and forth between these emotions, or experience two emotions simultaneously. Although Kübler-Ross's model is well known, it is not universally accepted. However, it is likely that at least some of the stages of grief will be experienced by most patients, and it can help to identify which of these emotions is being experienced so that you can respond appropriately.

Terminal diagnoses

Writing about patients with cancer, a Marie Curie report[57] cites much evidence that

> *'Good quality communication is capable of positively influencing a patient's emotional state, which, in turn, may have a positive impact on his or her health outcomes. The contrary also holds good: poor communication can lead to heightened anxiety and depression, which may then have a deleterious impact on the patient's health.'*

---

57 McDonald A for Marie Curie (2016) *A Long and Winding Road: Improving communication with patients in the NHS.* Available at: https://www.mariecurie.org.uk/globalassets/media/documents/policy/campaigns/the-long-and-winding-road.pdf (accessed February 2017).

It is not uncommon for patients with a terminal diagnosis to react with denial. This might involve questioning the diagnosis, or believing that test results are wrong. Think in advance about how you will handle such a reaction, so that you can manage it if the situation arises.

Terminal cancer patients and their families may have unrealistic expectations of cure. They might understandably be desperate for some hope, and plead for your help: 'Surely there must be some drug or treatment that will help? You must be able to do something, please.' It can be difficult in these circumstances to admit that there is nothing further that can be done in terms of treatment, but you must. However, never use the actual words 'There is nothing more that we can do', as it leaves patients feeling bereft and without hope. And in any case, even if there is no other treatment available, there are things that can be done, such as palliative care. (When explaining that active treatment is being withdrawn, stress the provision of 'symptom relief' or 'treatment for comfort' or other such terms, rather than using jargon such as 'palliative care'.) It is important that patients and their relatives do not feel hopeless.

The patient/family may have a strong emotional reaction when given bad news – such as anger, rage, crying, silence or denial – particularly if the news was completely unexpected. Such reactions can be difficult for practitioners to deal with. It is natural to want to reassure the patient and provide hope, but do not offer false reassurance or misleading optimism. Acknowledge the emotion being shown: 'I can see that you are angry and I realise that this must be very difficult for you.'

You may be asked very direct questions that you feel uncomfortable answering. Someone with a terminal diagnosis may ask, 'How long do I have left?' Or a young woman with cancer of the womb might enquire, 'Will I ever be able to have children?' They have asked the question because they want to know the answer. Humanely deliver honest responses – even when you feel awkward doing so. Their comfort must come before yours.

American surgeon Atul Gawande[58] believes that many doctors are not good at being honest with patients and telling them when treatments are unlikely to work. They are also very poor at estimating how much time terminally ill patients have left, overestimating on average by a factor of five. He recounts the story of a cancer patient at the end of his life, and how the professionals avoided talking honestly to him:

---

58 Gawande A (2014) *Being Mortal: Medicine and what matters in the end*. Toronto, ON: Doubleday Canada.

'We had no difficulty explaining the specific dangers of various treatment options, but we never really touched on the reality of his disease. His oncologists, radiation therapists, surgeons, and other doctors had all seen him through months of treatments for a problem that they knew could not be cured. We could never bring ourselves to discuss the larger truth about his condition or the ultimate limits of our capabilities, let alone what might matter most to him as he neared the end of his life. If he was pursuing a delusion [that treatment could restore the life he once had], so were we ... But admitting this and helping him cope with it seemed beyond us.'

Sometimes practitioners avoid facing these difficult conversations by focusing on things that are easier to discuss, such as physical symptoms. Avoid talking about the more difficult emotional needs of the patient – how they are feeling, their fear, or the impact of the disease on them – and you will be putting your needs above theirs.

Patients may not show their emotions in a clear and straightforward way. Yes, some will ask direct questions and talk about how they are feeling, but others will look shocked, or express disbelief, or say nothing, or speak but show no emotion at all. You will need to read the situation, without necessarily having overt clues to help you. Empathy will be called for. You may need to ask the patient open questions to help establish how they are feeling, and to help them to voice any concerns. If these opportunities to talk about emotions are ignored, the patient may be internally preoccupied with how they are feeling and unable to compute what you are telling them.

Reflect on how you might feel in their shoes. (Although also remember that patients are individuals and may not behave in the same way as you would. Their own circumstances, their personal resilience, and their outlook on life, will affect their reaction. Consider buying Dr Kate Granger's book[59] *The Other Side,* on her experiences as a doctor becoming a patient with a terminal cancer diagnosis. Her hope in writing it was that healthcare professionals could better understand what being the patient is really like and how their behaviours, no matter how small, can impact massively on the people they look after.) Where patients are shocked, confused or do not know their own feelings, you may have to help them explore these. Encourage clients to voice their emotions, but accept that some people may not want to. Never push anyone into areas of discussion where they feel uncomfortable.

The previous discussion assumes that the giving of bad news takes place at a time of your choosing, in a planned way. This may not always be the case. A patient may ask

---

59 All profits from the sale of the book are donated to the Yorkshire Cancer Centre.

you out of the blue, 'Do you think I might have cancer?' or some other direct question. The same rules still apply. Sometimes junior members of the healthcare team, such as students or healthcare assistants, may be asked such questions. If so, explain that you will need to get the clinician in charge to speak to them. It is not for you, but rather for the clinicians, to have such conversations with patients or relatives.

Sometimes healthcare staff have a facilitative role to play after bad news has been broken, in helping relatives to reach a consensus where various care or treatment options are available and there is no agreement as to what to do. It is not for you to push in a particular direction, but simply to provide the information and to use active listening, open questioning and clarifying to help them find their way through to an agreed position.

Cultural differences

Show respect for patients' religious and cultural beliefs. In some cultures, there is a tradition of protecting the patient from bad news such as a cancer diagnosis. Relatives might be keen to preserve that custom and could ask you not to reveal the bad news to the patient. While you must be aware of and respect cultural differences, remember that your primary responsibility is to the patient. Establish their preference as an individual rather than jump to a conclusion based on preconceived ideas about their cultural group – or relatives' wishes. Find out from them what and how much information they want to receive, and respect their wishes. Some cultures may adopt a collective approach to decision-making. If this concurs with the wishes of the patient, their view needs to be respected.

Dos and don'ts

- Do make sure that you've created the right setting, checking that there are sufficient chairs for everyone, for example.

- Don't delay informing the patient/relatives, even if you are dreading the encounter. They have a right to know, and it's your job to impart information sensitively. Research shows that most people want honest information delivered as close as possible to the time when the facts are known.

- Do consider involving a colleague in the meeting if they know the patient better or will be providing follow-up care.

- Don't overlook the value of body language. There are times when there are no words, but a sympathetic look or touch can speak volumes. (Research on touch has mixed findings: some saying that a touch on the hand was valued; others that it was unwanted.)

■ Do think about how to appear more approachable. Some practitioners believe that unfastening the jacket or lab coat can give a more open impression in difficult encounters.

Reflection

If you heard that you had a terminal condition, what questions would you want to ask your doctor? Make a list. Now think about the consultation with your doctor as if it were a business meeting. What would be on your agenda, as a patient? Could this information form a structure for how you could approach a consultation in which you as a practitioner have to break bad news?

Chapter 8: Written communication

From appointment letters to clients through to patient information leaflets, the written word is an important method of communication. Written information can be used to inform patients about their condition; to persuade them to adhere to their medication regime; or to reinforce what was said in a consultation. With a few simple writers' tricks, it is easy to communicate more clearly and concisely in writing.

Written information has many uses in healthcare, but is particularly valuable in reinforcing messages from a face-to-face consultation with a patient. However, it is only useful if it is well written and the information provided matches the material wanted by the reader. Poorly written, over-complex, unclear or ambiguous information is likely to be detrimental, causing possible confusion and anxiety for clients.

When we speak, it's usually a fairly spontaneous and instantaneous activity for which there is rarely a permanent record. Writing is generally a more considered act in which there is time to reflect on our choice and sequence of words, and an opportunity to review them in order to create a more exact, measured and deliberate (potentially permanent) communication. Writing is a different skill to speaking. People who are articulate when talking are not necessarily good at putting their words down on paper. However, writing is a skill that can be learned.

Writers must do without the visual clues such as facial expressions and body language that clarify and reinforce spoken messages. The written word is one-dimensional in comparison. As meaning must be conveyed purely with the words – without the added help of stress, intonation and non-verbal clues – it's vital that you choose those words carefully. They must convey your message clearly, succinctly and unambiguously. Too many printed materials rely on striking design for impact. Design can help attract interest, draw attention to important parts of the text, and help make patient information material easier to read – but good design is no substitute for good content.

Health literacy

Health literacy was defined by the World Health Organisation in 2015 as 'the personal characteristics and social resources needed for individuals and communities to access, understand, appraise and use information and services to make decisions about health'. Low health literacy is widespread, particularly in those aged sixty-five and over, black and minority ethnic groups, people in low-status jobs and those living in poverty. A study[60] assessing the readability (ease with which a reader can understand a written text) of healthcare information stated that poor health literacy:

> '… is associated with poor compliance with treatment and poor disease knowledge and may increase the risk of hospitalisation … Little is known about the degree of health literacy in the UK population, with small studies suggesting that inadequate health literacy is common.'

A more recent report[61] by the Royal College of General Practitioners (RCGP) quoted research by health literacy expert Gill Rowlands, which quantified the scale of the problem as follows: 'Forty-three percent of the English adult working-age population cannot fully understand and use health information containing only text. When numerical information is included in health information, this proportion increases to 61%.' This is concerning, as the same report concluded:

> 'Health literacy is needed for patients and the public to understand and act upon health information, to become active and equal partners in co-producing health, and to take control of their health to help to shape health environments and health services for themselves, their families and their communities.'

The authors found that improved health literacy brought about many benefits, including ensuring fairness and equity in the NHS; a more effective use of resources; and shared decision-making with patients. Conversely, low health literacy is associated with greater use of A&E and inpatient services, poorer

---

60 Fitzsimmons P, Michael B, Hulley J & Scott G (2010) A readability assessment of online Parkinson's disease information. *Journal of the Royal College of Physicians of Edinburgh* **40** (4) 292–296.

61 Royal College of General Practitioners (2014) *Health Literacy: report from an RCGP-led health literacy workshop*. Available at: http://www.rcgp.org.uk/clinical-and-research/clinical-resources/health-literacy-report.aspx (accessed February 2017).

self-management skills, and low uptake of preventative services such as breast screening and flu vaccination programmes – in the UK and in mainland Europe. As 90% of all face-to-face consultations in the NHS involve GP practices, GPs have a key role in improving their communication skills and tailoring information not only to clinical need, but also to patient health literacy levels. NHS managers have a role in ensuring that staff are aware of issues emanating from low health literacy.

It is natural for people with poor literacy to feel embarrassed, and this can prevent them from asking for clarification, and participating in discussions about the benefits and drawbacks of a procedure, or alternatives to it. This in turn can contribute to poorer health and poorer outcomes. It is believed that something as simple as a 'prompted question sheet' could be a useful tool for addressing health literacy issues and promoting interactive health literacy, by assisting communication between practitioner and patient. A list of possible questions, with a space for notes, could act to focus a consultation and to boost the number of questions a patient may have otherwise asked. Might this be something that you could produce for your workplace?

A similar concept to boost patient engagement is Ask Me 3, developed by the National Patient Safety Foundation and designed by health literacy experts. It encourages people to ask their healthcare professional three questions at the end of each appointment or consultation:

1. What is my main problem?
2. What do I need to do?
3. Why is it important for me to do this?

A British version, Ask 3 Questions, helps patients and service users to get the support they need to make informed decisions about their health and care. Based on research from Cardiff University and the Health Foundation, it encourages patients to ask:

1. What are my options?
2. What are the pros and cons of each option for me?
3. How do I get support to help me make a decision that is right for me?

Both of these programmes focus on the patient asking the questions, but it is essential that the healthcare professional can provide answers that the patient will understand.

'Teach back' is another useful technique in which practitioners check that they have been understood by asking the patient to paraphrase what they have heard. Teach back also improves patient recall, making them more likely to remember information given to them in a consultation.

Do not restrict yourself to spoken and written messages. Visual communication can be a helpful aid, such as showing patients multimedia presentations to help bring theoretical concepts to life.

It is essential that what you write is accessible to the wide range of audiences likely to be reading your materials. Use the practical advice in the rest of this chapter to help you achieve this.

Writing skills

To write effectively, start by thinking. This should be done well before you set pen to paper, or mouse to mat. Consider:

- **Audience:** Who are you writing for? An individual patient? A group of service users who share a particular medical condition? Another healthcare professional? How much do they know about the subject? How much time will they have to dedicate to it? Knowing as much about your reader as possible allows you to tailor the content.

- **Purpose:** What do you plan to achieve by writing? To convey information, such as facts about a medical procedure or test results? To persuade a patient to take a particular action, such as to adhere to their medication and exercise regime?

- **Message:** What do you need to communicate? What are your main and secondary points? What must you say and what can/should you leave out?

- **Medium:** What is the best way to communication your message? An email? A patient information leaflet? Sometimes the medium is obvious. If replying to a letter, you'll probably reply by letter. Always consider alternatives. Partway through lengthy written correspondence, you may recognise that it would be better to pick up the phone or meet face-to-face to resolve matters.

- **Tone:** How do you wish to come cross? Friendly and encouraging? Authoritative? Adopt a tone that is appropriate for the intended audience and the purpose of your writing.

Many of the healthcare practitioners I have spoken to say that they love the face-to-face work with patients, but dislike the writing part of their role and struggle to get words down on the blank sheet of paper or the clear computer screen. There is no need to feel that way. Writing is not difficult, and there are many techniques you can use to get you started. Regard writing not as a single process, but as a series of simple steps, each building upon the preceding one.

GAS-DECA: Seven stages of writing

Gather – Jot down ideas in any order.
Arrange – Group random ideas into clear themes.
Sequence – Organise themes into a logical order.

Draft – Produce a draft.
Edit – Polish the draft.
Consult – Show polished draft to the target audience.
Amend – Change draft in light of comments received.

This multi-stage approach can be used for any writing task: an important letter, a leaflet, a dissertation, an academic paper, a report for colleagues. Depending on the writing task, some steps may be omitted.

- **Gather:** Scribble down on a notepad all of your thoughts and ideas as they occur. Don't censor anything just yet. (It's easier to delete bad ideas later than to think only of good ones at the time.) This is just your starter for ten, not the finished product. It is a useful step even for a letter, as it can help ensure that you do not overlook something important when you come to write. (For a letter, it might take just a minute or so, whereas for a complex leaflet you might spend longer.) If you omit this stage and go straight to drafting, you may be concentrating on style and could miss important content.

- **Arrange:** Take your notes and organise related topics into groups. Incorporate new thoughts or ideas as they emerge. Evaluate ideas and delete initial thoughts that on reflection are irrelevant or unimportant.

- **Sequence:** Arrange your themed groups into a logical order – which may be chronological, alphabetic, or some other helpful sequence that will make sense to the reader. A structure should have emerged. You will find it easy to start writing now.

- **Draft:** Follow the above structure and fill in the detail. Concentrate on getting words down on paper. Ignore style and grammar for now. You can edit and refine your words later.

- **Edit:** Set your draft aside. Return to it later and read it with fresh eyes. Begin editing, looking out for jargon, repetition and any unnecessary words. If it's a letter or email, this might be a quick process (and one that you would only follow for important correspondence – routine correspondence can be drafted and then edited without a gap in between.) Documents with a long shelf life and/or wide circulation might merit more attention than a disposable email to a colleague.

- **Consult:** This step applies to patient information materials and such documents. Once you have a good working version of what you want to say, test-drive it on the intended audience. Ask what they think about its accessibility and readability. Is anything important missing? Might words, phrases or sections be changed to aid clarity? Are there any parts that are ambiguous? It is usually best practice to involve the target audience for patient materials from the outset, and not just at the end. Find out what information they would like to see included, and produce a draft that follows their guidance. At this stage, let the same group see and comment upon what you have produced. If necessary, involve clinical experts too.

- **Amend:** Carefully consider all of the feedback received, then amend your draft accordingly. This will ensure that your written material is the best that it can be.

Improving readability

If your writing is not readable, there is a good chance that it will not be read. What's the point of producing material that is ignored or cast aside in frustration? There is none. Readability is about how easy a piece of writing is to read and understand. This will, of course, vary across individuals depending on level of education and intelligence. But readability is really about the written material itself, rather than the reader. Readability concerns the vocabulary chosen, sentence length and construction, and design elements such as the visual look of text layout. Taken together, these factors can make a document an easy read – or a hard struggle.

Experts have devised various formulae that attempt scientifically and objectively to measure readability. Although his is not the first, Rudolf Flesch's mathematical readability formula devised in the 1940s is one of the better known. Text length, word length (based on syllables) and sentence length are weighted to create a readability score ranging from 0 to 100. The higher the number, the easier the text is to read. If I carry out the test on what I have just written, for example, this paragraph scores 53.7 on the Flesch scale (see below) – an assessment that this section of text is fairly difficult to understand.

Flesch scale

- 90-100: Very easy

- 80-89: Easy

- 70-79: Fairly easy

- 60-69: Standard

- 50-59: Fairly difficult

- 30-49: Difficult

- 0-29: Very confusing

The Flesch-Kincaid Reading Ease test followed in the 1970s, aligning the readability of text with what various American school grades would be expected to be able to read with ease. The Gunning Fog Index measures in a similar way to Flesch-Kincaid. It is based on sentence length and how many words of three or more syllables are used. The SMOG (Simple Measure of Gobbledygook) index is another option. A study[62] assessing the readability of online consumer-orientated Parkinson's disease information published in the *Journal of the Royal College of Physicians of Edinburgh* found that 'Flesch-Kincaid significantly underestimated reading difficulty' and that 'SMOG should be the preferred measure of readability when evaluating consumer-oriented healthcare material'.

You can purchase software to calculate the readability of your text, some word-processing programs come with it inbuilt, and there are also many free online calculators that can be used (for example, www.readability-score.com). Run a check on something you've written for patients to see how your writing scores. The following tips will help you to improve your readability score. Try them – then rerun the calculator to see if they have worked.

Create smaller chunks

One simple way to aid readability is to avoid great slabs of unbroken text, which can appear daunting and will make it harder to find the relevant information. Even short documents benefit from being divided into readable bite-size chunks. Try to use short paragraphs, each one containing a single idea. Break up text simply by using a combination of the following:

---

62 Fitzsimmons P, Michael B, Hulley J & Scott G (2010) A readability assessment of online Parkinson's disease information. *Journal of the Royal College of Physicians of Edinburgh* **40** (4) 292–296.

- **Bullet points:** These make long lists appear less daunting and ensure that listed items do not get lost in a sea of text.

- **Headings and subheadings:** These break up text and help readers navigate a document with ease.

- **Boxes:** In longer documents such as patient information booklets, boxes of text can serve the dual purpose of breaking up your text and drawing attention to the messages in the boxed section. Learning disability charity Mencap recommends 'story boxes' and 'fact boxes'.

- **Pull-quotes:** These are key phrases from the text that are used as a graphic element (usually reproduced in larger or distinctive typeface, or in a different colour). They are a good way of highlighting important information, as well as making text look more attractive and enticing.

Plain English

Plain English makes anything you write more readable for every audience – whether busy healthcare professionals, or people who struggle with the written word. The use of plain language is widely recognised as best practice because it makes written material easier to digest and less likely to be misunderstood. Also, plain English is easier to translate into other languages should you need to, and is more accessible for people whose first language is not English.

Plain English is not over-simplified 'Janet and John'-style writing. Rather, it is accessible, easy to read, clear, concise, unambiguous and unpretentious writing that uses the following:

- **everyday words** (try not to use words of three or more syllables; they are harder to recognise and read. Also avoid medical and technical jargon)

- **familiar words** (avoid Latin, foreign words and phrases, as unfamiliar words interrupt the flow and cause readers to struggle)

- **shorter sentences** (aim for 15-20 words. A 27-word sentence will be understood first time by just 4% of readers – the other 96% will have to reread it)

- **simple punctuation** (avoid colons, semi-colons and hyphens, as well as long sentences full of commas)

- **concise summaries where appropriate**

- **short, readable chunks of text**

- **active rather than passive verbs** (see p. 135)
- **the first and second person** where possible (I, you, we, rather than the hospital, the oncology unit).

Research has shown that common medical terms – such as the difference between the terms 'fracture' and 'break' – are sometimes misinterpreted or misunderstood by the public, both native and non-native English speakers – potentially leading to incorrect investigation and care. Words you might consider to be part of everyday vocabulary may not be understood, such as 'analgesia', 'biopsy' or 'chronic'. Researchers in the 1990s found that patients only understood just over a third of health professionals' commonly used terms. More recent research found that the term 'chronic' means 'persistent' to healthcare practitioners, but 'severe' to most laypeople. A report[63] by the Royal College of General Practitioners (RCGP) stated: 'Doctors can unintentionally use words that are unfamiliar to their patients, without realising that the meaning is not clear. Some concepts familiar and obvious to doctors may be alien to patients.'

Words carry connotations – 'drug' perhaps being associated with illicit substances, whereas 'medicine' is regarded as something that makes people better. Think about the vocabulary you use when writing for (and speaking to) a lay audience. Don't accept the first word that springs to mind. Consider whether your chosen word conveys your intended meaning and is the right one to use in the context.

For examples of healthcare jargon, and a free downloadable guide to writing medical information, take a look at the Plain English Campaign's website,[64] from where this example came: 'You should either take ciprofoxacin 1–2 hours before eating or drinking dairy products or avoid eating and drinking these products for four hours after taking ciprofoxacin.' Anything that requires reading more than once in order to be understood is not plain English.

A good healthcare example of plain English in action can be found on the Great Ormond Street Hospital website (www.gosh.nhs.uk). The writing style is friendly, accessible and clear. There is also a handy list of medical words with plain English explanations/definitions. For example, the condition achalasia, which is quite challenging to explain in simple terms, is defined on the site as follows:

'The oesophagus (food pipe) contains muscles which squeeze rhythmically to push food downwards. In achalasia, these muscles and the lower sphincter

---

63 Royal College of General Practitioners (2014) *Health Literacy: Report from an RCGP-led health literacy workshop.*

64 Plain English Campaign (2001) *How to Write Medical Information in Plain English.* Available at: http://www.plainenglish.co.uk/files/medicalguide.pdf (accessed February 2017).

(ring of muscle at the end of the oesophagus) do not work properly, so food cannot pass easily into the stomach to be digested.'

The site also has real-life stories that children, young people and families can relate to.

First person

Using words such as I, we, you and us makes writing more accessible. This is known as the first/second person (see Table 8.1). The third person (he, they, the NHS) was traditionally the default style in business/official communication, but its use makes text impersonal and distant: 'Patients must tell the Hospital when they have …'. Instead, write: 'Please tell us when you have …'. Practitioners use the first/second person when face-to-face with patients, so use it when you write too. Readability is improved when writing is close in style to the spoken word. Employ friendly, direct words such as 'I', 'we' and 'you'.

Table 8.1

First person	The writer	I, we, me, us, my, mine, our, ours
Second person	The reader	You, your, yours
Third person	A third party (the person or thing spoken about)	He/she, him/her, they/them, it, the hospital, the Trust, the NHS, the clinic

Writing 'I' when referring to yourself, and 'you' with reference to the patient, can help build relationships in a way that the more formal 'the hospital' or 'XYZ Trust' cannot. But while the first/second person style is often preferred, the third person is not banned. There will be occasions – for example, when you are stating your workplace's position or policy – that it may be inappropriate to use the first person. To do so would give the impression that it is your own personal policy. When writing 'we', be sure that you are expressing the agreed position of your workplace. 'I' is fine for your opinion; use 'we' when presenting your organisation's policy/position.

Active verbs

A simple trick to make your writing more succinct, direct and punchy is to use active verbs, as passive voice writing is more wordy and roundabout. The active voice is where someone does something:

'The chiropodist will see the client.' (6 words)
'The Radiology Department x-rayed the patient.' (6 words)

The passive voice is where something is done to someone:

'The client will be seen by the chiropodist.' (8 words)
'The patient was x-rayed by the Radiology Department.' (8 words)

As you can see from the above examples, the word order for passive sentences reverses. A couple of words may not make a big difference in a single sentence, but spread out across a longer text it does reduce word-count and aid readability.

Table 8.2

Active word order	Passive word order
1. Subject (the doer): chiropodist, radiology Department	1. Object
2. Verb (a doing word): to see, to x-ray	2. Verb
3. Object: the client, the patient	3. Subject

It is usually best to use the active voice when writing, but there are a few situations where the passive voice can be preferable. These include:

■ When you do not wish to admit liability, such as in the early stages of a complaint where culpability is not yet known. In such circumstances, it might be better to acknowledge that 'A mistake was made ...' (passive) rather than 'The Hospital made a mistake' (active). The active voice suggests that your organisation got it wrong, which may prove not to be the case, whereas the passive does not assign guilt.

■ When you do not know who or what the 'doer' is, such as in the following example, where the person who did the knocking down is unknown to the A&E staff: 'The casualty was knocked unconscious.'

■ When tact is required, such as when dismissing someone, reprimanding or rejecting them, or chasing unpaid bills: 'Your medicines remain uncollected' is softer than 'You have not collected your medicines.' The passive can be less accusatory or critical.

Poor literacy

Although very few adults in the UK are completely illiterate – unable to read or write anything – a significant minority are what is termed 'functionally illiterate'. That means that their literacy levels are at or below what would be expected of an 11-year-old child. While they can understand short, straightforward written material on familiar topics, reading information from unfamiliar sources, or on unfamiliar topics such as medical issues, could prove very difficult for them.

Over 5 million adults[65] in England are functionally illiterate. Rates for other parts of the UK are similar. Add to that people who are dyslexic (around 10% of the population[66]), plus the even larger percentage of the population who struggle to understand numerical information (such as their chances of being affected by an adverse side effect from a drug), and you begin to see the scale of the problem. Even well-educated people may not understand common numerical ways of explaining risk likelihood, such as 'a one-in-ten chance' or 'a 10% chance'. Verbal descriptions, such as 'common' and 'likely' even left medics confused, according to research. However, some ways of explaining magnitude do resonate with people, such as 'That's the equivalent of the Albert Hall/Wembley Stadium at full capacity' or 'It's equal to seven jumbo jets.'

Look out for potential signs of functional illiteracy, which might include:

- taking a long time to write one's name and address
- use of block capitals when not required
- reading slowly
- claiming to have forgotten to bring reading glasses
- offering to complete the paperwork later, at home.

Adults can be ashamed about poor literacy skills and too embarrassed to admit that they struggle. If you believe that a patient may be functionally illiterate, be sensitive when it comes to giving written information for them to take away. Make sure they leave a consultation with full understanding, as they may be unable to consult the leaflets later.

Don't forget that some people may be unable to read due to their medical condition, and other formats such as audio and audiovisual will need to be

---

65 National Literacy Trust (2017). Available at: http://www.literacytrust.org.uk (accessed February 2017).
66 Dyslexia Action (2016). Available at: http://www.dyslexiaaction.org.uk/page/about-dyslexia-0.

provided as an alternative to written materials (with subtitles and/or British Sign Language (BSL) translations where necessary). Consider alternative written formats too, such as Easy Read.

Easy Read

'Easy Read' is a way of communicating to people with learning disabilities. To see examples of healthcare leaflets created in Easy Read, go to www.easyhealth. org.uk. Easy Read is not the straight translation of a document into easier-to-understand 'plain English'; it is a complete rewriting that emphasises the essential information and does away with much of the background detail. Pictures support the meaning of the simplified text. Someone with a learning disability may be able to understand an Easy Read document independently; others will need a carer or healthcare professional to talk it through so that they can understand it and make decisions if necessary. (Easy Read materials can also be helpful for other audiences, such as people who are not fluent in English and people who have had strokes.)

When producing Easy Read materials, involve people with learning disabilities and follow these guidelines published by the Department of Health England:[67]

- **Length:** Keep it below 20-24 pages. If it exceeds 24 pages, split it over more than one publication. In longer documents, consider stating at the beginning that the reader doesn't have to read the whole publication and can ask for support reading it. Include contents and an index in longer documents.

- **Sentences:** Keep them short and simple – no more than 10 to 15 words. Each sentence should have just one idea and one verb. Make sentences active not passive.

- **Words:** If you must use a difficult word or idea, highlight it (possibly in a different colour), then define it using easy words (in the next sentence, not as part of the same sentence). Delete unnecessary words: 'take this medicine for 14 days' rather than 'for a period of 14 days'. Use the same word or form of words when referring to the same thing, rather than a variety. Avoid acronyms and abbreviations. If you must use them, include a glossary explaining them and any difficult words.

A font point size of 14 or 16 is recommended, and a bigger size still for headings. Break text into small chunks, as long tracts may not be understood. Highlight

---

67 Department of Health (2010) *Making Written Information Easier to Understand for People with Learning Disabilities*. Available at: http://www.inspiredservices.org.uk/Government%20 EasyRead%20Guidance.pdf (accessed February 2017).

important points using bullets, boxed text and emboldened text, but avoid using too many sets of bullet points close together.

Easy Read dos and don'ts

- Do say 'half' (not 50%), 'a quarter' (not 25%), and '1 in 5' (not 20%)

- Don't say '67%', say '67 out of 100'.

- Don't use percentages unless you have to. If you must, write 'percent' (rather than the symbol %).

- Do use whole numbers (7 percent, not 6.8 percent).

- Don't spell out numbers (one, four) – express them in figures: 1, 10, 100. However, for millions say 3 million, 20 million.

- Do format dates as follows: Monday 16 January 2017. Do not abbreviate the year to '17.

- Don't use the 24-hour clock, as it may confuse. Pictures of analogue or digital clocks can help explain the time.

- Do highlight important dates at the beginning, such as the date that a response is needed to a letter, or the date of an appointment.

It is not only people with a learning disability who struggle with numbers. The independent charity National Numeracy's 2016 YouGov poll found that only one in four people could fully understand the sugar information in a nutrition label. Gill Rowlands, Professor of General Practice, Institute of Health and Society at Newcastle University, and founder of Health Literacy Group UK, says on the National Numeracy website (www.nationalnumeracy.org.uk) that patients

> '... need to be able to understand and manage numbers for many areas of health. We need these skills to stay healthy (such as knowing how to eat healthily, get the right exercise, have safe levels of alcohol drinking), prevent illness (such as understanding our own risk of diabetes or deciding whether cancer screening is right for us), and manage illness (such as knowing how and when to take our tablets) ... Health literacy is people's knowledge and ability to obtain, understand and apply health information. Clearly numeracy is key because so much health information is in numbers. Without numeracy skills people will not be able to make sense of the information they are given.'

Professor Rowlands advises that healthcare staff must take extra time to ensure they have explained health issues involving numbers well enough for patients to understand. This includes such things as explaining medications, talking through decisions about whether to have a flu jab or take a cancer screening test. You may find that patients value visual ways of being presented with numerical information – such as pie charts and infographics – to help everyone to understand your message.

Easy Read images

Pictures, drawings, photographs and other images are a key component of Easy Read (but use only one illustration style throughout the document). Each main idea needs both words and pictures, although there is no need to use a picture for every sentence: too many pictures against one short paragraph can be confusing. Place pictures next to the accompanying text to aid understanding, ensuring that the link between the pictures and text is clear. Chosen images must be easy to understand and should help explain the text. Position pictures to the left of the text, and ensure images are as big and clear as possible (using high-resolution images or photographs). Colour pictures are preferable, and the use of words in pictures should be kept to a minimum.

Dyslexia

Dyslexia is a learning difficulty that can cause problems with reading, writing and spelling. The charity Dyslexia Action defines it as a 'specific learning difficulty', which means it causes problems with certain abilities used for learning, such as reading and writing. Unlike a learning disability, intelligence isn't affected. Around 10%[68] of people in the UK has some degree of dyslexia – although it is not the same for everyone, and can range from mild to severe.

Dyslexia is lifelong problem that can present daily challenges. Someone with dyslexia may understand spoken information, but have difficulty with written information. They may read and write very slowly; confuse the order of letters in words; put letters the wrong way round – such as writing 'b' instead of 'd'; have poor or inconsistent spelling; and find it hard to carry out a sequence of directions.

The British Dyslexia Association (BDA) has produced advice to ensure that written material takes into account the visual stress (text appearing distorted, blurry or moving) experienced by some dyslexic people (www.bdadyslexia.org.uk). The advice facilitates ease of reading for dyslexic people, but much of it applies to other groups too – so even if your materials are not aimed specifically at people with dyslexia, you may find that ease of reading is improved for many groups.

---

68 Dyslexia Action (2016). Available at: http://www.dyslexiaaction.org.uk/page/about-dyslexia-0.

Dos and don'ts

- Do use matt paper, which is thick enough to prevent text or images on the other side from showing through.

- Don't use glossy paper or white backgrounds, which can appear too dazzling.

- Do use cream- or soft-pastel-coloured paper – and dark-coloured text.

- Don't use green and red/pink, as these are difficult for colour-blind people.

- Do use a plain, evenly spaced sans serif font such as Arial and Comic Sans in point size 12-14.

- Don't use narrow newspaper-style columns. Keep lines of text to around 60 to 70 characters, using a line spacing of 1.5.

The BDA also advises avoiding underlining and italics, as they can tend to make text appear to run together. Use bold instead. Avoid block capitals, even in headings. For headings, use a larger font size in bold. Boxes and borders are effective for emphasising text. Use left-justified text (with a ragged right edge). Avoid long, dense paragraphs. Don't start a sentence at the end of a line. Give instructions clearly, using simple steps. Avoid double negatives. Flow charts are a useful device for explaining procedures. Pictograms and other graphics can help dyslexic readers to locate information within the text. Lists of dos and don'ts are useful for highlighting key information. It is worth looking at the BDA's guidance (which can be found at www.bdadyslexia.org.uk), as it also contains very helpful information on preparing electronic documents for text-reading software.

Inclusive language

If you use non-inclusive language when writing (and speaking), you will alienate a portion of your audience. They may fixate on your inappropriate language and stop reading your message. This is counterproductive, so always try to use inclusive language.

Dos and don'ts

- Don't refer to females over 18 as 'girls' – they are women.

- Do only mention gender ('lady doctors' or 'male nurses') if their gender is relevant to the point you are making.

- Don't use language that excludes women – words or expressions like: 'The man in the street'; 'telephones manned by'; 'layman', and so forth.

- Do use gender-neutral terms whenever possible: chair (or chairperson). Avoid feminine forms such as 'care home manageress'.

- Don't write 'he/his/him' when you are writing about people in general. Avoid gender-exclusive language by pluralising; rephrasing the sentence to avoid the word him altogether; or using neutral terms such as 'patient' or 'client'.

- Don't use the word 'black' in a negative way: 'black day', 'blacken the name of', and so on, as it could cause offence to non-white people.

- Do use terms such as 'people with a disability' or 'people who are blind' rather than 'the disabled' or 'the blind' in order to recognise the person before the disability.

Now let's look at some of the written materials healthcare practitioners may need to produce.

Patient information materials

Considerable evidence from many sources suggests that patients regard written patient information materials such as leaflets, booklets and factsheets very positively, as they present a range of benefits, including:

- reinforcing spoken health messages

- supplementing what was said in a consultation

- providing a resource to refer to at a later date, thus reminding the patient of information that might otherwise have been forgotten

- being able to boost or refresh understanding of what a healthcare practitioner said, once away from the stresses of the clinical consultation

- increasing patient's knowledge and understanding of an issue or condition

- providing information to help patients prepare for an event such as an operation or hospital stay

- helping patients feel informed and confident about taking decisions about their care and treatment

- answering patients questions and queries

- sharing information with other family members.

If patients are to value and trust patient information materials, the content must be clear and concise (while not omitting anything important); neither over-complex nor patronising; accurate, credible and authoritative; up to date and relevant; and unbiased. Every piece of patient information will be unique, but here are some broad areas that you may need to include:

- information about a particular condition
- signs and symptoms
- managing the condition and self-help
- possible tests and treatments and their risks and benefits
- details of a procedure
- side effects and complications
- uncertainties and conflicting opinions
- text addressing concerns and providing reassurance if appropriate
- challenges to common fears and misconceptions
- anonymised real-life case histories
- everyday analogies that aid patient understanding
- facts and figures presented in a way that makes sense to the reader – prevalence, survival or complication rates, for example
- sources of further information and support.

Leaflets created to inform – 'Your diabetes questions answered' or 'The benefits of a low-salt diet' – can benefit from the Q&A (questions and answers) format. Such a format is easy to write and to read. A question is also a good device for the front cover – 'Want to know more about healthy eating?' (Never ask a question in a headline unless readers will answer it with a 'yes'.)

Different audiences may have very different requirements, so bear this in mind when writing patient information materials. For example, the storybook format is good for pre-sevens; and information in comic-strip form can appeal to children, but be a turnoff for teens. The Patient Information Forum[69] recommends the use of short sentences in a logical order when writing for children and young people; simple vocabulary; graphics to illustrate rather than numbers (which can be confusing); and the presentation of facts in a short and punchy way, such as 'Did you Know?' This is good advice, but arguably applies to a wider audience and not just to materials aimed at children and young people.

69 The Patient Information Forum (2014) *Guide to Producing Health Information for Children and Young People*. Available at: http://www.pifonline.org.uk/wp-content/uploads/2014/11/PiF-Guide-Producing-Health-Information-Children-and-Young-People-2014.pdf (accessed February 2017).

Dos and don'ts

- Do consider using a 'highlights' section in longer documents to flag up key information early on (such as side effects or any risks).

- Don't forget to consider including a Q&A section that directly addresses patients' frequently asked questions.

- Do include a date on the publication where appropriate so that patients know how recent the guidance is.

- Don't use overlong words and sentences or complex language structures. Stick to plain English.

- Do ensure readers know what you are saying at first reading, as they are unlikely to reread in order to work out your message.

Patient correspondence

Letters

A letter to a fellow professional may well be characterised by a brief, concise style that gets straight to the point: 'I am writing to you enclosing Mrs McTavish's test results. Please acknowledge receipt and let me know if you have any queries.' Busy professionals need to quickly understand your purpose in writing, and what (if anything) you expect from them by way of action. There are circumstances where you should ask for confirmation that your communication has been received, such as when sending test results or other important information. Never assume that because you sent something, it was received. Complete the feedback loop by asking for confirmation so you receive the necessary assurance that your important information has reached the recipient safely.

Letters to patients may be quite businesslike too if they are simple and transactional: 'Your six-monthly follow-up appointment is now due. Please contact the surgery to arrange a suitable time.' Reflect on the purpose of a patient letter, because you may need to provide more information than the bare minimum. Reassurance or further detail may be required: 'You will be pleased to hear that your bowel-screening test results are normal. You do not need to be tested for the next three years, although if you experience any of the following symptoms before then, please contact your GP ...'

Patients may find long letters daunting, so if you need to convey a lot of information, consider whether you might supplement the letter with a more detailed enclosure – such as an accessible patient information leaflet, a list of Q&As or a fact sheet. Be sure to refer to enclosures in any covering letter, explaining what you have enclosed and why. Invite the patient to contact you if anything remains unclear.

The Royal College of General Practitioners stated,[70] 'Increasingly, patients are sent copies of clinic letters; they struggle to understand these and this may be a source of frustration and confusion.' If you are enclosing correspondence that a patient may not understand, ensure that your covering letter provides a plain English explanation.

Email

Email has been around for years, and most of us use it at work and socially, although the NHS has been slow to use it for patient communication. According to a 2016 article in the *British Medical Journal*,[71] this is believed to be because staff fear that the ease of using email would mean that clients would be more likely to correspond excessively, resulting in staff being unable to cope with the size of their inboxes. Consequently, posted mail is still used in many parts of the NHS.

Where email is used, it may not be being used appropriately. The BMJ article cited above said: 'Doctors are using email without referring to guidelines, with potential patient safety and medicolegal implications'. The authors advise that to preserve confidentiality, patients should be asked to consider which household members have access to an email account if it is to be used to correspond about health matters. Where patients say that they wish to communicate with you about their treatment via email, ensure that they explicitly consent, understand and accept the risks with this form of communication – including understanding that correspondence to an account such as Gmail or Hotmail may not be secure and will not be encrypted. Also ensure that such correspondence complies with your organisation's information governance standards.

Always take sensible precautions to protect patients' confidentiality, or you could end up paying a high price. In 2016, Chelsea and Westminster Hospital NHS Foundation Trust, which runs a sexual health clinic, was fined £180,000 after revealing sensitive personal data – the email addresses of hundreds of users of an HIV service. The Information Commissioner's Office (ICO) found there had

---

70 Royal College of General Practitioners (2014) *Health Literacy: Report from an RCGP-led health literacy workshop*. Available at: http://www.rcgp.org.uk/clinical-and-research/clinical-resources/health-literacy-report.aspx (accessed February 2017).

71 Sowerbutts H & Fertleman C (2016) How best to use email with patients. *BMJ* **352** (8040) 87.

been a serious breach of the Data Protection Act, which was likely to have caused substantial distress. The clinic allowed patients with HIV to receive test results and make appointments by email – and to receive an occasional newsletter. A small number of people on the newsletter mailing list did not have HIV. An error, in which email addresses were wrongly entered into the 'to' field instead of the 'bcc' ('blind copy correspondence' field – where other recipients' email addresses cannot be seen), meant that newsletter recipients could see each other's email addresses, 730 of which contained people's full names.

An ICO investigation found the Trust had made a similar error in 2010, when a member of staff in the pharmacy department sent a questionnaire to 17 patients in relation to their HIV treatment, entering emails in the 'to' field instead of the 'bcc' field. Take great care not to make such a mistake. The fines imposed for breaching confidentiality in this way can be substantial, but the damage to trust can be even more costly.

Email is not a suitable medium to convey complex or sensitive information to a patient (nor is a letter), so always consider whether a face-to-face meeting is more appropriate than a written communication. Where email is a suitable channel, give such correspondence the same care and attention as any other written communication, whether initiating contact or replying. Many of the rules for letter-writing apply.

Chapter 9: Communicating with colleagues

Good communication is crucial to clinical effectiveness and to the safe and compassionate care of patients. From succinct and accurate transmission of patient information to other members of the clinical team, through to proper record-keeping, effective communication is essential. This chapter also looks at how to communicate effectively in groups and teams comprising other health and social care professionals.

Effective patient-centred care requires healthcare professionals to communicate not only with the patient, but also with each other (about the patient). The more collaborative approach that has been brought about through better integration of health and social care should help ensure the best outcome for the patient. However, health and social care is a complex landscape, and working across multidisciplinary teams requires exceptional communication. During their care, a patient may see a wide variety of professionals in different organisations, across a range of professional groups or a multiplicity of specialisms. Risk is elevated for that patient, as they are seen by various professionals and pass through different health and social care organisations, and there is a real danger that things can go wrong. Good communication amongst the professionals can avert problems and ensure safe and effective care.

Record-keeping

Written clinical records are one of the principal ways of recording and communicating information across the clinical team, with a view to ensuring safe and effective practice and good patient outcomes. Registered healthcare professionals learn how to write records (such as care plans, clinical notes, birth plans and observation charts) during their training, but that's no guarantee of being naturally a good record keeper. Writing on the BMJ Careers website in 2014, Wedad Abdelrahman and Abdelrahman Abdelmageed stated that:

> *'… medical record-keeping is often given a low priority. Notes are often poorly maintained and sometimes patient notes are not readily available. It is common to find illegible entries, offensive comments, and missing information, and there is often inconsistency between entries by doctors, nurses, and midwives.'*

Other researchers, too, have identified many common failures, so there may be scope for improving how you communicate through your healthcare records, and it is certainly worth reflecting periodically on how you are writing up patient records. Not all members of the healthcare team are given adequate training in record-keeping: unregistered healthcare assistants, particularly those working outside of the NHS, may have received little training in this important area.

With the growth in litigation in healthcare, a worrying development is in the number of lawyers, rather than clinicians and communicators, who are teaching record-keeping. Such an approach can result in clinicians believing that the purpose of a record is to protect them should litigation ensue. While undoubtedly a well-written and comprehensive record will indeed do that, a defensive motivation is unhelpful. The purpose of a record is to document patient care and to share that information with colleagues so that they can provide excellent continuity of care when you are not there.

Good records matter

- Good records are central to patient safety. While a comprehensive clinical record may not in itself improve patient care, a poorly written or incomplete record increases the risk of error, leading to poorer outcomes for patients.

- Communication is improved between healthcare professionals and across the wider team.

- Communication is improved with patients and relatives. By practitioners referring to the notes, patients get a consistent message rather than confusing and contradictory accounts.

- Partnership in care is facilitated if patients and carers can understand records.

- If there is a serious adverse incident or near miss, the record can be valuable to assist organisational learning and improvement.

■ Records will be scrutinised should you ever find yourself before your professional regulator; a coroner's inquest or Fatal Accident Inquiry; facing criminal proceedings; an ombudsman investigation; or subject to a complaint from a patient.

Most courts and disciplinary panels (workplace and regulatory) take the view that if you didn't write it down, the care that you say you provided didn't take place. As a Fitness to Practise panellist for the Nursing and Midwifery Council (NMC), I chaired panels that removed nurses from the Register because they were unable to prove that they provided the care or treatment that they claimed to have given. Had they kept full and accurate contemporaneous records, they may still be practising today. Don't let that happen to you. Recognise the importance of good record-keeping – both for you and your patients – but always keep the patient's interest as your first priority when you write them, rather than thinking of them as evidence that might be used in your defence should anything go wrong.

It is always best to write up your notes as close as possible to the time that the care was provided, as a contemporaneous record will be more accurate than one written up later from memory. If you cannot complete your notes at the time, make sure that when you do catch up, you record the time the care was given, as well as the time your notes are being written.

English NHS record-keeping guidance[72] for staff states: 'Health care professionals must develop communication and information sharing skills as accurate records are relied on at key communication points, especially during handover, referral and in shared care'. The Nursing and Midwifery Council Code[73] requires that nurses must 'communicate effectively, keeping clear and accurate records'.

Common failures

Record-keeping need not be onerous, time-consuming or difficult, yet still practitioners sometimes get it wrong and make fundamental communication mistakes. Learn from these common errors:

■ **Lack of specificity** – Rather than 'Fluid intake 600mls' (timeframe unspecific), write 'Drank 400mls at 9.00am, and a further 200mls at 11.15am'.

---

72 NHS Professionals (2016) *CG2 Record Keeping Guidelines*. Available at: http://www. nhsprofessionals.nhs.uk/Download/CG2%20-%20Record%20Keeping%20Guidelines%20V5%20 2016.pdf (accessed February 2017).

73 NMC Code (2015) *Professional Standards of Practice and Behaviour for Nurses and Midwives*. Available at: https://www.nmc.org.uk/globalassets/sitedocuments/nmc-publications/nmc-code.pdf (accessed February 2017).

■ **Failure to document key information** – such as relevant information gleaned from telephone calls and conversations, or details of problems that have arisen. If you include too much irrelevant detail, there is a risk that the critical information that you have documented may be overlooked because your record is unnecessarily long.

■ **Lack of detail and clarity** – 'Mr Smith unhappy. Didn't want to eat, but perked up when daughter visited' is unclear. What is meant by 'unhappy' and how did this manifest itself? Providing more detail can aid clarity: 'Mr Smith feeling down and didn't want to get out of bed this morning. Persuaded to get up, wash and dress for breakfast. Ate two slices of toast and drank two full cups of tea. Mood improved when daughter visited at 11.00am. Ate all his lunch at 1.00pm.'

■ **Omissions** – If you record that a patient is in pain, also record what you did in response. If you provide any care, write it up. If you decide that something is not required, make a note explaining why. If a patient has any special needs, make a note of them.

There is no national standard for record-keeping, and great variation can be found across the NHS. Even use of a unique patient identifier (the NHS Number in England and Wales, the CHI – Community Health Index number – in Scotland) on the record is open to variation, with some hospitals still preferring to use the hospital number. Refer to your workplace policy and guidelines. Regardless of your seniority, or whether you are using paper or electronic recording systems, observe the standards that your employer expects and your profession requires.

Dos and don'ts

■ Do keep it factual and clear – with dates and times (using the 24-hour clock) where applicable, and your signature at the end (with your name and designation printed).

■ Don't use generalities. Keep it specific. Include measurements where applicable.

■ Do write legibly if not using electronic patient records, using neat handwriting in non-erasable black ink. Make it understandable too, exercising care when using acronyms and abbreviations that others may not be familiar with.

■ Don't record personal opinions and judgements about the patient or their relatives – stick with neutral descriptions and facts; avoid speculation; and never use insulting, discriminatory or subjective statements. A good test is whether you would be happy for the patient to read what you have written.

- Do involve the patient or carer if possible, and use language that they can understand.

- Don't omit anything important – including explanations, if you do decide not to do something.

- Do ensure that if you need to delete, amend or alter records because of a factual error, the correction is clearly shown as an alteration. Record the date and time that the amendment was made, and your name and signature.

Reflection

Do you know what your employer expects from you in terms of record-keeping? When did you last read the policy or guidelines? What about your regulator or professional body, if you are a regulated practitioner? Are you confident that you comply with all aspects of the relevant policies? Do your colleagues comply? If not, what have you done about it? Have you ever asked colleagues for feedback on your documentation? Might there be value in doing so?

Avoiding 'never events'

Effective communication can prevent 'never events', and in this way it can protect patients from harm. The NHS defines a 'never event' as a wholly preventable incident with the potential to cause serious patient harm or death. Examples of never events are: wrong patient procedures; wrong site surgery; retained instrument post-operation; and wrong route administration of chemotherapy.

A report[74] analysed 9 of the 57 wrong patient, wrong site or wrong procedure surgical never events that occurred in a single year in the NHS in England and Wales. Of the non-technical skills identified as contributing to the errors, communication failures were found to be a contributory factor in many of the cases examined, with examples of failures in staff-to-patient communication; communication between teams; and communication between front-line staff and management. The report cites the case of a young cancer patient, who had a temporary abdominal spacer inserted in the wrong side. The abbreviation 'RT' was used in his notes, but it meant different things to different clinicians involved in his care. To the oncology team, RT referred to radiotherapy; to the surgeons,

---

74 Department of Health Human Factors Reference Group (2012). *DH Human Factors Group Interim Report and Recommendations for the NHS*. Available at: http://chfg.org/policy-research/dh-human-factors-group-interim-report-and-recommendations-for-the-nhs/ (accessed February 2017).

it was an abbreviation for right side. In another case, a cancer patient had the wrong lymph node removed. The term 'groin' was interpreted differently by the oncologists and the surgeons, which led to the confusion.

The report concludes that in these and other cases, better communication could have prevented these never events from happening. For example, the simple act of briefing the team before surgery could have played a part in reducing the likelihood of error. Briefing is such a quick and simple communications technique, in which information is exchanged in order to ensure shared understanding, but it can prevent these catastrophic occurrences. Communication is two-way, and a briefing should also empower colleagues to speak up about concerns, or simply to ask questions for clarification. In the cases examined in the above document, had there been an opportunity to stop and ask, 'Can I just check that …?' errors could have been avoided. The learning from this is clear. The group behind the report concluded that a key learning point to emerge from their work was 'the significant role that good handover and communication has to play in delivering safe care'.

A more recent analysis[75] of 23,658 medical malpractice claims and law suits between 2009 and 2013 involving patient harm was undertaken in the United States by CRICO (a division of the Risk Management Foundation of the Harvard Medical Institutions, Incorporated). It found that at least one specific breakdown in communication occurred in 30% of cases, contributing to patient harm. Of all high-severity injury cases, 37% involved a communication failure. Communication errors involved face-to-face conversations, electronic exchanges, errors in writing or interpreting the patient's clinical record, and systems failures in sharing information such as test results.

Dos and don'ts

- Do be alert to any ambiguity when writing up notes.

- Don't forget that if ambiguity could arise, your notes must be sufficiently detailed to allow only one possible meaning. This is especially important when using abbreviations and acronyms that could be misunderstood.

- Don't use general terms such as 'groin'. Always be as specific as possible, including 'left'/'right' or 'upper'/'lower'.

- Do ensure that training is multidisciplinary where appropriate and possible, so that there is consistency in terminology and abbreviations within your organisation.

75 CRICO Strategies (2015) *Malpractice Risks in Communication Failures 2015 Annual Benchmarking Report*. Available at: https://www.rmf.harvard.edu/Malpractice-Data/Annual-Benchmark-Reports/1-Request-CBS-Report-PDFs (accessed February 2017).

- Don't make assumptions if there is insufficient detail in patients' notes – check out the missing facts.

- Do document any differences in meaning of clinical terms across different teams that could lead to error, and ensure that this is shared.

It is tempting to believe that frequently used medical terms are commonly understood, but that may not be the case. Various terms may mean different things to different teams within the same workplace, as seen in the previous examples. Further examples include 'PID' (meaning 'prolapsed intravertebral disc' for one team; 'pelvic inflammatory disease' for another) and 'TOF' ('tetralogy of Fallot' for some clinicians; 'tracheo-oesophageal fistula' for others). To help avert confusion, many healthcare workplaces have developed a published glossary of acceptable abbreviations, with a full explanation of the terms. Has yours?

Clinical handover

Whether you call it handover, a change of shift report or a nursing report, it's accepted that this exchange of clinical information is a fundamental communication opportunity upon which patient safety rests. Handovers give the care team time to discuss a patient's treatment, to share problems or concerns, and to check that everyone knows exactly what's happening on the ward/ residential home. The handover can ensure that tasks are neither missed nor repeated unnecessarily, and that a consistent approach is taken with patients and relatives – by sharing what they have been told, so there is no contradictory information provided.

An inpatient will experience at least three shifts of different staff daily, with handover providing an opportunity for things to go wrong if the communication exchanged is inaccurate or insufficiently focused. A week in hospital represents a minimum of 21 potential opportunities for adverse events arising from an inadequate handover – more if the patient is moved to different wards, where further handover will be required. The World Health Organization[76] observed:

'The hand-over (or hand-off) communication between units and between and amongst care teams might not include all the essential information, or information may be misunderstood. These gaps in communication can cause serious breakdowns in the continuity of care, inappropriate treatment, and potential harm to the patient.'

---

76 WHO (2007) Communication during patient handovers. *Patient Safety Solutions* **1** (Solution 3).

Writing in 2004, Professor Sir John Lilleyman, then Medical Director of the National Patient Safety Agency, went further: 'Handover of care is one of the most perilous procedures in medicine, and when carried out improperly can be a major contributory factor to subsequent error and harm to patients.'[77]

There is no set format or national standard for handover, although most healthcare organisations will have a clinical handover policy that covers:

- who is required to attend handover – including any non-clinical staff
- who will lead clinical handover
- the designated time and venue for handover
- structure for what and how information at handover is communicated, recorded and retained.

Many organisations provide a standardised communications framework or template to ensure consistency. Handover typically involves sharing the following pertinent information about a patient:

- patient name, age and date of admission
- diagnosis and treatment plan (including important details such as nil-by-mouth, for example) and resuscitation plan if applicable
- information about the patient – such as whether they need help with eating, washing or using the toilet; whether they are diabetic; any allergies; and whether they have specific communications needs (because they are deaf or blind, for example)
- for newly admitted patients, the circumstances that led to admission
- changes in the patient's condition or management plan – any improvement/deterioration (or risk of deterioration), and results from any assessments or investigations
- tasks yet to be completed that need to be picked up by the new shift – such as dressings that need to be changed or checks that should be made. These should be in priority order and delegated to specific people
- what the patient/relatives have been told
- any follow-up arrangements, such as likely discharge, follow-up tests, referrals or future appointments.

---

77 BMA Junior Doctors Committee (2004) *Safe Handover, Safe Patients: Guidance on clinical handover for clinicians and managers*. Available at: https://www.bma.org.uk (accessed February 2017).

It's important to limit handovers to essential information, to ensure that priority areas do not get lost in a mass of unimportant information. Handover is a two-way process, so allow time for questions to be asked. There must be no ambiguity or uncertainly after your shift has finished. If you are on the receiving end of a handover, ensure that you have absolute clarity and ask questions if you are at all unsure.

Read-back is often used in handovers, as a useful check that everything has been understood. The handover recipient makes a note of the oral handover information given, and then reads it back to the provider. Confirmation that it has been understood correctly is given, or clarification and correction is provided where misunderstandings have arisen.

Many hospitals have a policy of performing handovers at the bedside. There is evidence to suggest that staff and patients alike value this. Bedside handover is a tangible demonstration to the patient that communication about their care is taking place. This in turn boosts confidence, makes them feel that staff are focused on them and their specific needs, and helps build rapport. Confidential information that is not appropriate for sharing in this way is written in the notes and shared with colleagues after the bedside part of the handover.

Good bedside handover arrangements that involve patients bring many benefits. The National Nursing Research Unit at King's College London,[78] for example, found that effective bedside handover:

■ supports communication between nurses and other healthcare professionals about a patient's health, care plan and progress, and improves safety and efficiency of care, including communication about medication (it works because staff communicate and interact in a structured way)

■ helps inform patients (and their relatives) about their care (so long as the information provided is understandable to them) and who is caring for them, and to interact with staff and ask questions

■ creates opportunities for patients to find out information and to be involved in care decisions that affect them

■ allows nurses time to observe and listen to patients, and improves the quality of information about patients.

---

78 Kings College London (2012) What are the benefits and challenges of 'bedside' nursing handovers? *Policy+* **36**. Available at: https://www.kcl.ac.uk/nursing/research/nnru/policy/By-Issue-Number/Policy--Issue-36.pdf (accessed February 2017).

However, bedside handover is not without challenges. Accurate documentation is essential to support effective bedside communication, to ensure that information is not overlooked, and to enable staff absent at handover to access vital information. It is also essential to inform patients and their families about what bedside handover is, what they can expect, how families can be involved in the process, and how privacy and confidentiality are protected. The King's College National Nursing Research Unit report suggests that this information is provided to patients in writing, so they can digest fully what bedside handover means for them.

Dos and don'ts

If undertaking bedside handover:

- Do be clear about what information can and cannot be shared at the bedside.

- Don't forget to involve the patient and, if appropriate, their relatives in the handover.

- Do remember to introduce colleagues if they are not known to the patient.

- Don't regard an oral bedside handover as a substitute for written notes: it is a supplement.

- Do give patients written information on how bedside handover works.

Communicating in groups

Today's healthcare is often provided by a multidisciplinary team. Communication within that team may involve team or case meetings, as well as handover. Communicating within a group is very different to a one-to-one interaction. People who are confident in smaller conversations can feel quite intimidated in the formality of a meeting or in a group of professionals – especially if others are more senior.

In group settings, it is common for participants to adopt different roles and styles. Where there is no appointed chair, someone might assume that role and lead or facilitate the meeting. There will be creative people who play the part of idea-generators; there will be cautious individuals; those who like to point to the flaws and shortcomings in other people's arguments; enthusiastic types; people who prefer to come in at the end and provide a summary of key points; and many other types too.

Reflection

What is your personal style when contributing to a group discussion? Does it vary depending on the group? Are you confident or shy? Do you talk too much or too little? Reflect on your contributions and on whether you could be a more effective participant. Think of a group participant whom you admire, and analyse what makes their contributions so effective.

When communicating in a group, have an idea beforehand of the key points you wish to contribute, then create opportunities to make them (if such opportunities fail to materialise naturally in the course of the meeting). Some people think that the best way to make an impact in a group is to have the loudest voice and the longest contributions. They are wrong. Keep your offerings succinct, focused and relevant. Always choose quality over quantity.

Meetings can only be effective if people listen to each other; failure to do this is discourteous and unprofessional. Preparation is important too. If there's paperwork, read it. If not, think about topics that are likely to be discussed and have a few ideas lined up and ready to be presented. Don't dominate the meeting, even if you have a lot to say. Encourage others where necessary.

Report writing

Reports are a key tool for providing information, often to enable a decision to be made by your colleagues, bosses or Trust/health board directors. Few people enjoy writing them, as the task can appear quite daunting. However, it need not be a chore. Good report writers understand what readers need. When you're the reader, what would you say are the hallmarks of a well written report? Most of us seek:

- brevity and succinctness

- logical order

- clear, well-argued proposals with supporting data

- clear identification of risks, benefits and resources

- unbiased reporting, with counter views presented and evaluated

- clear recommendations or next steps, with alternatives if appropriate

- visual messages such as graphs, charts and tables that can convey complex information quickly and simply.

Key ingredients

Many organisations have a standard structure for reports. Common headings/sections include:

- Purpose – the reason for the report: to seek funding for a new MRI scanner.
- Summary – a paragraph summarising the contents/key points of the report.
- Background – information about the background or summarising the history of that issue/concern. Each report should be self-contained; do not assume that a previous report on the subject will have been read or remembered.
- Main body – methods used; facts and figures; discussion of the issues; results; options and alternatives; pros/cons.
- Conclusions.
- Recommendations – excessive or irrelevant information will obscure your recommendations, so keep them succinct.
- Financial and/or other implications (such as an equality impact assessment, communications implications and so on).
- Glossary and appendices.
- Bibliography/references.

Not every report will contain all of these elements. Select what to include according to the convention in your organisation and the requirements of the report you are writing.

When asked to write a report, get a good brief so you know what is expected, cover all of the pertinent issues, and produce the right report first time. Ask for:

- a summary of why the report is needed
- key points or areas you need to cover
- issues to be avoided (if any) – it may be that some areas will be covered in another report that is being produced, or there are sensitivities about certain issues
- details of people you should consult with (if any) or documents you should refer to when creating your report
- required length. Some authors wrongly believe that a long report is more impressive. Reports should be as short as possible, while including sufficient

information to enable readers to understand the recommendations made or the conclusions reached

■ a deadline.

Dos and don'ts

■ Do differentiate between fact and opinion.

■ Don't use jargon and avoid abbreviations where possible – if you must use some, provide explanations.

■ Do use an appendix for information that is useful but not directly pertinent to your conclusions.

■ Don't omit contrary views, or your report will appear one-sided.

■ Do strike a sensible balance between what must go in and what can be left out.

■ Don't forget to include a summary in long reports, containing enough for readers to understand the thrust of the full document without having to read it.

Staff memos

The memo is an internal document, usually brief, often issued to a number of people at the same time, to inform staff of new information (such as policy changes, new procedures, or new staff); to remind them of or to update them on policies or standing operating procedures; or to notify them of events (such as staff meetings or seminars). It can be an important communication tool in situations such as busy wards or care homes, where staff are on rotas and there may be no opportunity to sit down with everyone to share information.

A memo comprises:

■ Heading: 'Memorandum' or 'Memo' in large type.

■ Date: the date of issue.

■ To: the name of the person/people to whom it is issued – Dr Joe Bloggs, or All staff in Ward 10.

■ From: the name of the writer or sender (and job title if appropriate).

■ Subject: a short, factual and informative description which flags up urgency where necessary e.g. URGENT: Use of XYZ Oxygen Cylinders – patient safety concerns.

■ Body text: your message. Begin with a short paragraph explaining why you are sending it and why recipients need to read it: 'This memo is about recent incidents concerning XYZ oxygen cylinders that requires your urgent attention. Please read it and inform your line manager that you have read it by October 12th'. Use bold, italics or underlining to draw attention to key text that needs to stand out.

Email

The NHS has been slower than many other organisations to adopt widespread use of email for patient communication, although it is used for colleague-to-colleague contact. Because emails can be written and sent quickly and without cost – unlike a letter (which must be printed, placed in a stamped/franked envelope, posted etc.) – it is tempting to simply fire them off to all and sundry without much thought. This would be unwise. Email is a useful tool, but you should apply the same level of thought to an email as to a letter. Recognise that it can be easier to create a negative relationship using email than with face-to-face or even telephone communication.

If your colleague asks you five questions, provide five answers in your reply, because an incomplete response will generate a further email. Pre-empt additional queries too: it will save time in the long run by concluding the correspondence sooner. If an email is becoming too long, consider a short, covering email with a more detailed response attached: Dear Mike, Thank you for your 15 questions on the Trust's paternity leave policy. I have addressed each in turn in the attached document. Please contact me if you need further clarification.

Always be careful about what you write in an email. Freedom of Information legislation means that emails you have written about someone (even internal ones) may be available to that named person. But regardless, it is unprofessional and unwise to make personal or injudicious comments about anyone in an email (or any other medium) – and such remarks would likely be in breach of your professional code. If a subject is sensitive, delicate or open to being misconstrued, email may not be the best medium.

Information security

Don't send confidential or sensitive patient information or commercially sensitive information to the wrong person. Always check the 'To' line before pressing send, and ensure that you use an encrypted network. Encryption is automatic from one NHS email address to another – accounts ending in @nhs.net are part of the secure national email service that enables the safe and secure exchange of sensitive and patient identifiable information within the NHS and with local/central government. Emails from/to @hotmail, @gmail, @yahoo, @btinternet, @doctors.net, and so on, should not be considered secure. Always apply the relevant protective markings to emails and attachments.

Dos and don'ts

- Do open with a salutation – Dear Hamish, Dear Dr Gupta – and end with your contact details.

- Don't use capital letters (except in a subject heading), as they signify shouting in email etiquette. Also, people with a visual impairment find capitals harder to read.

- Do include an explanatory subject line so it's clear what your message is about. This also enables the recipient to assess your email's priority and to file and retrieve it easily. Also mark it for information/action/urgent action as applicable.

- Don't 'reply to all' unless everyone on the original list needs to see your reply.

- Do resist the temptation to copy something too widely when initiating an email. Save your colleagues' time by copying-in only those people who need or want your communication.

- Don't use your personal email to communicate with colleagues, or your NHS email to communicate with friends.

If you are out of the office, set up your account to send an automatic out-of-office message that includes the date when you will return and the name and contact details of the person to contact in your absence. This will communicate to the sender that you are away, so that they can chase up the matter with a colleague if it is urgent.

Communication outside work

Healthcare practitioners are required to uphold the reputation of their profession, but some get into hot water by failing to recognise and manage their communications outside of work.

We all have many different personas: healthcare professional, parent, friend, partner, sibling … and our behaviour naturally varies according to the role we are playing. The kind of banter we have with friends may be of a type that we rightly recognise as being inappropriate were it to take place with a patient. However, there are some behaviours that are inappropriate for a regulated healthcare professional in any circumstance – even when they are off-duty. It is difficult to be specific, as context is everything.

A mechanic enjoying an evening of excess after work, whilst still wearing his overalls branded with his employer's name, may be an idiot, but he's not necessarily bringing his trade into disrepute. However, a nurse in the same circumstances could well be, especially if uniform is involved. Such behaviour would communicate a negative message about the individual, but it could also damage their employer and the reputation of the wider profession.

Like the police and the legal profession, registered healthcare professionals are expected to observe high standards of behaviour – higher than ordinary citizens. There is also a professional code of conduct to uphold, and breaches could lead to removal from the relevant healthcare register and resultant loss of livelihood. The standard of behaviour expected extends to off-duty time too.

Rowdy, drunken behaviour has always been an issue to consider, but more recently social media has emerged as an area where certain standards of behaviour are expected. Most professional codes single it out for mention. The General Medical Council's (GMC) online guidance *Good Medical Practice* (2013), for example, says: 'You should remember when using social media that communications intended for friends or family may become more widely available.' The Nursing and Midwifery Council's (NMC's) Code says: 'Use all forms of spoken, written and digital communication (including social media and networking sites) responsibly, respecting the right to privacy of others at all times.' Even where professional codes do not explicitly mention social media, caution is required. For example, the NMC's Code states that nurses and midwives must '[m]aintain effective communication with colleagues', but NMC guidance stresses that working co-operatively with colleagues includes communicating in an appropriate way when using social media.

The GMC says that the 'standards expected of doctors do not change because they are communicating through social media rather than face to face'. Even with the proviso that 'all opinions expressed are my own', you may still land in trouble if comments are inappropriate or breach patient or workplace confidentiality. Careless communication could cost you your job – particularly if you identify yourself as a healthcare professional when posting.

Reflection

The NMC advises: 'It is important to consider who and what you associate with on social media. For example, acknowledging someone else's post can imply that you endorse or support their point of view. You should consider the possibility of other people mentioning you in inappropriate posts. If you have used social media for a number of years, it is important to consider, in relation to the Code, what you have posted online in the past'.

Consider your own private postings on Facebook, Twitter, Instagram, Flickr and other social networks, blogs and chatrooms. Have you ever posted anything that would cause you embarrassment were your boss, colleagues, patients or the media to see it? Think about your online image and how it reflects on your professional standing. Does it enhance it or diminish it?

Problems can sometimes arise when colleagues are also social media friends, such as Facebook friends. In such circumstances, the boundaries between professional/ work discussion and social interaction can become blurred. Even if privacy settings are such that you believe posts cannot be viewed beyond your friendship group, there is still scope for a post to be inappropriately shared by someone within that group.

The following social media communications are likely to get you into trouble:

- sharing confidential information about patients, colleagues or your employer
- using publicly accessible social media to discuss patient care – even if it is with the patients themselves
- posting pictures of patients and clients receiving care
- posting inappropriate comments about patients – even if no names are mentioned
- harassing or victimising someone, or attempting to prevent or discourage someone from raising concerns
- posting complaints about colleagues or your workplace
- making gratuitous, unsubstantiated or unsustainable comments about individuals online
- using social media to build or pursue relationships with patients or service users
- encouraging violence or self-harm, hatred or discrimination

- posting material online without declaring any conflicts of interest related to the post, such as financial or commercial interests in healthcare organisations or pharmaceutical and biomedical companies.

Approaches from, or contact with patients or ex-patients through social media channels must never be accepted. Contact and engagement with patients or ex-patients must always be through appropriate workplace/healthcare channels. It is generally recommended that Facebook friend requests from current or former patients should not be accepted. Professional boundaries must be maintained. Should a patient contact you through your private social media profile, explain that yours is a professional relationship and refer them to the appropriate way of contacting you or your organisation. The British Medical Association (BMA) advises:

> 'Given the greater accessibility of personal information, entering into informal relationships with patients on sites like Facebook can increase the likelihood of inappropriate boundary transgressions, particularly where previously there existed only a professional relationship between a doctor and patient. Difficult ethical issues can arise if, for example, doctors become party to information about their patients that is not disclosed as part of a clinical consultation. The BMA recommends that doctors and medical students who receive friend requests from current or former patients should politely refuse and explain to the patient the reasons why it would be inappropriate for them to accept the request.' [79]

Social media is not all doom and gloom, and there are real benefits for healthcare professionals in using it appropriately. It can be used to:

- engage in healthcare, professional and policy discussions

- establish professional networks in the UK and globally using sites such as LinkedIn

- facilitate patients' access to appropriate information about their health and supportive services

- engage with the public about relevant healthcare issues – such as the Twitter accounts of ambulance community first responders promoting the benefits of learning CPR

- gain information about current issues in healthcare – by using trusted websites such as NHS.uk

---

79 British Medical Association, London (2011) *Using Social Media: Practical and ethical guidance for doctors and medical students*. Available at: http://www.gmc-uk.org/static/documents/content/Doctors_use_of_social_media.pdf (accessed February 2017).

- share information with colleagues and learn from them on online communities – using blogs and internet forums aimed at particular professional groups – such as doctors.net.uk and the BMJ's doc2doc.

Many healthcare practitioners have well-respected Facebook pages and Twitter accounts, which attract many followers. In Scotland, where I live, the Chief Medical Officer, Chief Nursing Officer and Chief Executive of the NHS all tweet regularly, as do many medical and nursing directors of health boards. So although there are pitfalls to using social media, don't let that put you off using a very valuable communications tool. Just be sensible when using this medium to communicate.

Each chapter of this book has demonstrated how effective communication produces good outcomes – whether for patients, practitioners or healthcare organisations. The evidence is clear. A Marie Curie report[80] summarised it neatly: 'It is safe to conclude that a clear link has been established between better quality communication and positive health outcomes. This link is evident across a variety of conditions and settings.'

Better communication is in your hands. You have the ability to improve, and this book has given you practical ideas. But reading alone is not enough, as Gwen van Servellen, Professor Emeritus at the University of California's School of Nursing, said in her book *Communication Skills for the Health Care Professional: Concepts, Practice, and Evidence*:

> *'Just reading about communication is not sufficient, however. Despite the abundant literature on communication and therapeutic response modes, communication knowledge and skills cannot be learned from textbooks alone. The critical test of providers' competency is how they put these principles and skills into practice with patients.'*

So, make the commitment to do something positive on the communications front right here, right now. There is no excuse for inaction – and no need to put it off until another day. Get on with it today, and become the 'good communication champion' in your workplace. Spread the word to colleagues and put it into practice yourself. Lend your copy of this book to someone on your shift. Plan a learning event around some of the reflective exercises in each chapter. You'll find work so much more rewarding when the whole team is fully engaged with improving communications!

---

80 McDonald A for Marie Curie (2016) A *Long and Winding Road: Improving communication with patients in the NHS*. Available at: https://www.mariecurie.org.uk/globalassets/media/documents/policy/campaigns/the-long-and-winding-road.pdf (accessed February 2017).

Finally, encourage your colleagues to commit to the following top ten communications tips, which will help ensure that they too are powerful patient-centric communicators.

Communications top ten tips

1. Regard everyone as an individual, and tailor your communications to meet their specific needs.

2. Use appropriate body language yourself, and 'read' and react appropriately to others' body language.

3. Look at the speaker, listen actively, and show that you are listening.

4. Always use plain English – when speaking and writing – using jargon only if you are confident that it will be understood.

5. Always address the patient rather than their relative, carer or translator.

6. Use written materials to reinforce your spoken message if necessary, but ensure everything is readable and in an accessible format.

7. Keep clear, factual (dates, times, measurements), relevant and contemporaneous patient records – including what you did, what you did not do, and why.

8. Use clarifying questions to check that you understand, and also check that you have been understood.

9. Present healthcare information in a clear, understandable, neutral and balanced way so patients can weigh up the pros and cons and reach an informed decision on next steps.

10. Identify early on interactions that may escalate into unpleasantness, and intervene to try to avert a difficult situation, but use good communication skills to defuse tension if tempers flare.

References

Action on Hearing Loss (2017) *Communication Rights for People who are Deaf or Hard of Hearing*. Available at: https://www.actiononhearingloss.org.uk/supporting-you/communication-support/i-am-a-service-provider-looking-for-communication-support/communication-rights-for-people-who-are-deaf-or-hard-of-hearing.aspx (accessed February 2017).

Archer J, Regan de Bere S, Bryce M, Nunn S, Lynne N, Coombes L & Roberts M (2014) *Understanding the Rise in Fitness to Practise Complaints from Members of the Public*. 21 Jul. Camera with Plymouth University.

Baile WF, Buckman R, Lenzi R, Glober G, Beale EA & Kudelka AP (2000) SPIKES – A Six Step Protocol for Delivering Bad News: Application to the patient with cancer. *Oncologist* 5 302-311

Berry D (2007) *Health Communication: Theory and Practice*. Maidenhead: Open University Press.

Bleich SN, Bandara S, Bennett WL, Cooper LA & Gudzune KA (2014) Impact of non-physician health professionals' BMI on obesity care and beliefs. *Obesity* 22 2476–2480.

How to Communicate Effectively in Health and Social Care © Pavilion Publishing and Media Ltd and its licensors 2017.

BMA Junior Doctors Committee (2004) *Safe Handover, Safe Patients: Guidance on clinical handover for clinicians and managers*. Available at: https://www.bma.org.uk (accessed February 2017).

British Medical Association (2011) *Using Social Media: Practical and ethical guidance for doctors and medical students*. Available at: http://www.gmc-uk.org/static/documents/content/Doctors_use_of_social_media.pdf (accessed February 2017).

Bruder Stapleton F (2000) My name is Jack. *Journal of the American Medical Association* **284** (16) 2027.

Care Quality Commission (2016) *2015 Inpatient Survey: Statistical release*. Available at: http://www.cqc.org.uk/sites/default/files/20150822_ip15_statistical_release_corrected.pdf (accessed February 2017).

Cooke NW, Wilson S, Cox P & Roalfe A (2000) Public understanding of medical terminology: Non-English speakers may not receive optimal care. *Journal of Accident and Emergency Medicine* **17** 119–121.

CRICO Strategies (2015) *Malpractice Risks in Communication Failures 2015 Annual Benchmarking Report*. Available at: https://www.rmf.harvard.edu/Malpractice-Data/Annual-Benchmark-Reports/1-Request-CBS-Report-PDFs (accessed February 2017).

Crystal D (2010) *The Cambridge Encyclopaedia of Language* (3rd Edition). Cambridge: Cambridge University Press.

Davies M (2015) Fat doctors 'should be struck off for setting a bad example to their obese patients', weight-loss expert tells NHS chief. *Mail Online* **6 July.**

Department of Health (2010) *Making Written Information Easier to Understand for People with Learning Disabilities*. Available at: http://www.inspiredservices.org.uk/Government%20EasyRead%20Guidance.pdf (accessed February 2017).

Department of Health Human Factors Reference Group (2012) *DH Human Factors Group Interim Report and Recommendations for the NHS*. Available at: http://chfg.org/policy-research/dh-human-factors-group-interim-report-and-recommendations-for-the-nhs/ (accessed February 2017).

Dyslexia Action (2016) Available at: http://www.dyslexiaaction.org.uk/page/about-dyslexia-0.

Fitzsimmons P, Michael B, Hulley J & Scott G (2010) A readability assessment of online Parkinson's disease information. *Journal of the Royal College of Physicians of Edinburgh* **40** (4) 292–296.

Gawande A (2014) *Being Mortal: Medicine and what matters in the end*. Toronto, ON: Doubleday Canada.

General Dental Council (2013) *Standards for the Dental Team 2013*. Available at: http://www.gdc-uk.org/Dentalprofessionals/Standards/Documents/Standards%20for%20the%20Dental%20Team.pdf (accessed February 2017).

General Medical Council (2011) *The State of Medical Education and Practice in the UK*. Available at: http://www.gmc-uk.org/State_of_medicine_Final_web.pdf_44213427.pdf (accessed February 2017).

General Medical Council (2013) *Good Medical Practice*. Available at: http://www.gmc-uk.org/guidance/good_medical_practice.asp (accessed February 2017).

GPhC (2010, reprinted 2012) *Standards of Conduct, Ethics and Performance*. Available at: https://www.pharmacyregulation.org/sites/default/files/standards_of_conduct_ethics_and_performance_july_2014.pdf (accessed February 2017).

Granger K (2012) *The Other Side.*

Harrahill M (2005) Giving bad news gracefully. *Journal of Emergency Nursing* **31** (3) 312–314.

HCPC (2016) *Guidance on Conduct and Ethics for Students*. Available at: http://www.hpc-uk.org/assets/documents/10002c16guidanceonconductandethicsforstudents.pdf (accessed February 2017).

Kings College London (2012) What are the benefits and challenges of 'bedside' nursing handovers? *Policy+* **36**. Available at: https://www.kcl.ac.uk/nursing/research/nnru/policy/By-Issue-Number/Policy--Issue-36.pdf (accessed February 2017).

Kübler-Ross E (1969) *On Death & Dying: What the dying have to teach doctors, nurses, clergy and their own families*. New York: Scribner.

McCartney M (2014) Fat doctors are patients too. *BMJ* **349**. Available at: http://www.bmj.com/content/349/bmj.g6464 (accessed February 2017).

McCulloch P (2004) The patient experience of receiving bad news from health professionals. *Professional Nurse* **19** (5) 276–280.

McDonald A (2016) *A Long and Winding Road: Improving communication with patients in the NHS*. Available at: https://www.mariecurie.org.uk/globalassets/media/documents/policy/campaigns/the-long-and-winding-road.pdf (accessed February 2017).

McEwen A and Kraszewski S (Eds) (2010) *Communication Skills for Adult Nurses*. Maidenhead: Open University Press.

Montague E, Chen P, Xu J, Chewning B & Barrett B (2013) Nonverbal interpersonal interactions in clinical encounters and patient perceptions of empathy. *Journal of Participatory Medicine* **5** e33.

Mulley A, Trimble C, Elwyn G (2012) *Patients' Preferences Matter: Stop the silent misdiagnosis*. King's Fund.

Muñoz MA (2014) *Does Bilingual Make you Smarter?* Available at: https://www.britishcouncil.org/voices-magazine/does-being-bilingual-make-you-smarter (accessed February 2017).

National Literacy Trust (2017) Available at: http://www.literacytrust.org.uk (accessed February 2017).

NHS England (2015a) *Accessible Information: Implementation plan*. Available at: https://www.england.nhs.uk/wp-content/uploads/2015/07/access-info-imp-plan.pdf (accessed February 2017).

NHS England (2015b) *NHS Chaplaincy Guidelines 2015: Promoting Excellence in Pastoral, Spiritual and Religious Care*. Available at: https://www.england.nhs.uk/wp-content/uploads/2015/03/nhs-chaplaincy-guidelines-2015.pdf (accessed February 2017).

NHS Professionals (2016) *CG2 Record Keeping Guidelines*. Available at: http://www.nhsprofessionals.nhs.uk/Download/CG2%20-%20Record%20Keeping%20Guidelines%20V5%202016.pdf (accessed February 2017).

NICE (2015) *Violence and Aggression: Short-term management in mental health, health and community settings*. Available at: https://www.nice.org.uk/guidance/ng10 (accessed February 2017).

NMC Code (2015) *Professional Standards of Practice and Behaviour for Nurses and Midwives*. Available at: https://www.nmc.org.uk/globalassets/sitedocuments/nmc-publications/nmc-code.pdf (accessed February 2017).

Parliamentary and Health Service Ombudsman (2010-11) *Listening and Learning: The ombudsman's review of complaint handling by the NHS in England*. Available at: http://www.ombudsman.org.uk/__data/assets/pdf_file/0019/12286/Listening-and-Learning-Screen.pdf (accessed February 2017).

Parsons SR, Hughes AJ & Friedman ND (2016) 'Please don't call me Mister': patient preferences of how they are addressed and their knowledge of their treating medical team in an Australian hospital. *BMJ Open*.

Plain English Campaign (2001) *How to Write Medical Information in Plain English*. Available at: http://www.plainenglish.co.uk/files/medicalguide.pdf (accessed February 2017).

Reid M, McDowell J & Hoskins R (2011) Breaking news of death to relatives. *Nursing Times* **107** (5) 12–15.

Royal College of General Practitioners (2014) *Health Literacy: Report from an RCGP-led health literacy workshop*. Available at: http://www.rcgp.org.uk/clinical-and-research/clinical-resources/health-literacy-report.aspx (accessed February 2017).

Sowerbutts H & Fertleman C (2016) How best to use email with patients. *BMJ* **352** (8040) 87.

Taylor SP, Nicolle C & Maguire M (2013) Cross-cultural communication barriers in health care. *Nursing Standard* **27** (31) 35–43.

The Learning Disability Partnership Board in Surrey. *The Hospital Communication Book*. Available at: https://www.mencap.org.uk/sites/default/files/2016-06/hospitalcommunicationbook.pdf (accessed February 2017).

The Patient Information Forum (2014) *Guide to Producing Health Information for Children and Young People*. Available at: http://www.pifonline.org.uk/wp-content/uploads/2014/11/PiF-Guide-Producing-Health-Information-Children-and-Young-People-2014.pdf (accessed February 2017).

Warnock C (2014) Breaking bad news: issues relating to nursing practice. *Nursing Standard* **28** (45) 51–58.

WHO (2007) Communication during patient handovers. *Patient Safety Solutions* **1** (Solution 3).

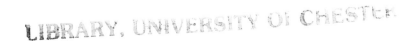